DIY AGELESS SKIN

Make Your Own Anti-Aging Skin Care Products for Less Money and Better Results

Robyn Phelan

ISBN-13: 978-1514603567
ISBN-10: 151460356X

The URLs for websites referred to in this book were functional and relevant at the time of publishing. The author and publisher are not responsible for the websites and, therefore, cannot guarantee that a site will remain available or that its content will remain relevant or appropriate.

CONTENTS

0
INTRODUCTION

Anti-aging skin care is a multi-billion dollar industry that preys on both men and women's desperation to get rid of their brow lines, crow's feet, and turkey necks. Beauty product manufacturers know that any formulations offering potential "age-defying" benefits can be sold for obscene prices because consumers have shown that they're willing to pay obscene prices. The mere hope of recapturing their youth compels them to spend ungodly sums of money on cosmetics, even after disillusionment sets in. New products are coming out all the time, and the current "next big thing" seems to rekindle their faith in skin care science, despite any past grievances. The unfortunate truth, however, is that most commercial anti-aging products don't work, and they never will. If they did, every baby boomer would have the complexion of a twenty-year-old, and cosmeceutical companies would lose recurring income from consumables. "The money is in the treatment, not the cure," as the saying goes.

When it comes to wrinkles and sagging skin, prevention is the best approach, but if it's too late for that, there are a few corrective measures that one can take to improve the appearance of his or her skin. If commercial anti-aging products have left you unimpressed with their results or lack thereof, then you'll be pleased to know that by taking matters into your own hands, you'll have the potential to reverse or reduce the signs of aging, both inside and out. Making beauty products from scratch isn't as expensive as you might think, and it doesn't take much time once you've found the combinations of active ingredients that work best for your skin. While the do-it-yourself (DIY) approach to ageless skin care is a trial-and-error process that can be frustrating at times, the rewards are undeniable:

1) You'll save money in the long run (there are some upfront costs). Advertising, marketing, attractive packaging, and functional but unnecessary ingredients such as pigments and fragrances contribute to the high cost of anti-aging products. You can dramatically reduce what you spend by making your own stuff. And with homemade products, a little bit tends to go a long way, so you may find that you don't get to the bottom of the jar as quickly as you may have in the past with a comparable store-bought item.

2) You don't have to worry about your favorite products being discontinued by their manufacturers. Your own products will become your new favorites, and never again will you have to settle for subpar alternatives.

3) You can control the amounts of active ingredients. One of the reasons that commercial anti-aging products don't work is that they contain active ingredients in amounts that are too small to be effective. Most of the ingredients are inactive, and their collective purpose is to form a lotion, cream, or serum to facilitate the spreading and absorption of the active ingredients. A manufacturer can add a single drop of an active ingredient, and that would be enough to put it on the label but not enough for it to make an impact. When you make your own products, you decide what to put in them and how much. (Do keep in mind, though, that some ingredients may cause adverse side effects if present in concentrations above a certain level, so be sure to research any potential issues that a substance may have before committing to its use.)

4) You can exclude unwanted ingredients that may be irritating, toxic, or unnecessary. One of the primary motivations of many DIY skin care hobbyists is to avoid ingredients that are of questionable safety.

5) Formulations that you create yourself may be higher in quality and more effective than over-the-counter (OTC) or prescription products. Your recipes will be tailored to your skin's needs, which is especially important if you have sensitive skin or dermatological conditions that may be aggravated by the mediocre skin care products that are commonplace in drug stores.

6) You can make your concoctions in small batches when needed so that you're always guaranteed a fresh product. Skin care merchandise may sit on the shelves for months or years, and some labels don't show an expiration date, so you don't really know if the products are safe to use or if their active ingredients have decomposed.

7) It can be a lot of fun. Once you experience the "wow factor" of something that you developed on your own *that actually makes a difference in your skin*, don't be surprised if this undertaking blossoms into a hobby, or even a business. You might also find yourself replacing all of your commercial soaps, hair care products, and makeup with your own superior creations.

Given the above, I should emphasize that this is **not a recipe book**. I'm reluctant to include recipes because everyone's skin chemistry is different, and what works for me might yield disastrous results for you. I also love to tweak recipes to make them better, so whatever formulas I would have included in this book when I wrote it wouldn't necessarily be the latest and greatest iterations by the time you discovered it and started reading. I believe that it's more constructive to tell you what you need to know about anti-aging skin care before embarking on your DIY adventure because there are plenty of mistakes to be made (ask me how I know). Having said that, I do share my personal lotion recipe through my website, but only for readers of this book. Please visit **robynphelan.com** for more information.

Again, DIY skin care is a trial-and-error process, and it's not uncommon to experiment with several recipes for a particular type of product before discovering a formula that works best for you. One way to make that discovery sooner rather than later is to purchase some artisanal skin care products that have the ingredients that you're interested in so that you can see how you like them. For example, if you're drawn to the benefits of hemp oil, you might purchase sample quantities of different hemp oil products such as lotions and soaps, as well as the pure oil itself. This may seem like an expensive first step, but it's a lot cheaper than purchasing all of the ingredients to make these products yourself, only to find out that you're not satisfied with them. In that case, you'd have unused portions of ingredients that, for sanitary reasons, cannot be returned for a refund and then sold to someone else.

So now you might be wondering, "Why don't I just buy other people's homemade products and call it a day?" There's nothing wrong with that, but if one of your goals is to save money on beauty products, then be aware that these other people are selling their wares to make a profit (not that there's anything wrong with that, either). As such, retail prices are several times higher than what it actually costs to make the products, and once you know what's in them, it can be much less expensive to make them on your own time and dime.

"But I won't know the recipes," I can hear you saying. Unlike commercial products with a laundry list of ingredients, artisanal skin care products that have only a few key ingredients aren't difficult to reverse-engineer. Certain ingredients can only be used in certain quantities (normally a percentage of the product's total weight, not including packaging) when co-existing with certain other ingredients. Therefore, you can research what quantities are appropriate for the type of product (e.g., lip balm), and piece together a working recipe. You can also swap some ingredients for others that are similar.

Suppose that you find a recipe that calls for sweet almond oil, but you don't like this oil for whatever reason. You can usually substitute another oil in the same quantity without botching the recipe. You could even substitute two or three oils for the original one, as long as the total amount of oil remains the same because using too much or too little can lead to poor texture and consistency.

Hopefully, I haven't made DIY skin care seem more complicated than it really is. If you're good at adapting food recipes to suit your palate or dietary needs, then you already have more than enough skill to make your own cosmetics and toiletries that may be better for your skin than anything else you've ever used. A happier, younger-looking you is not beyond reach if you're willing to keep an open mind and put forth a bit of effort.

DIY Ageless Skin, however, is about more than extolling the virtues of making your own products; it's about encouraging you to take a proactive, whole-body approach to aging. There's only so much that topical anti-aging treatments can do to make you look younger or delay the onset of fine lines and wrinkles. Since aging occurs internally as well, you can slow this process by addressing factors within your control, such as your diet, lifestyle, and hormonal balance. Nutrient deficiencies, sleep deprivation, chronic stress, and a host of other issues often manifest as ailments of the skin, hair, and nails. Therefore, becoming healthy on the inside is likely to result in positive changes in the way you look and feel. Since an entire book could be written about each of several subtopics in this one, my discussion of anti-aging skin care is meant to provide information in enough detail to be useful, while giving you a foundation for further research. My goal is for you to come away from this book feeling empowered with the knowledge to either sustain a youthful complexion well into old age or make life-changing improvements in the appearance of mature skin.

1

MY "DIY AGELESS SKIN CARE" PHILOSOPHY

Simplicity and minimalism are major themes in my life, and they have made their way into my skin care regimen. After nearly three decades of using store-bought cosmetics and personal care products, I became fed up with both the quantity and quality of the products that I was using. On the rare occasion that I found a "perfect" product, I'd later have to spend time and money looking for a suitable alternative because the manufacturer decided to either discontinue the product or sell a "new and improved" version, in which the only "improvement" that I could see was an increase in the company's profit margin on account of using cheaper ingredients. In one case, the new formula was so different from the old one that I wondered how they could get away with selling it under its original name.

With the industry trend being to cut production costs while raising prices and lowering quality, I decided to take matters into my own hands. The switch from commercial to (mostly natural) homemade products has been not only enlightening, but also age-defying. I'm still amazed at how much of a difference certain botanical oils have made in my complexion. I no longer feel the need to wear foundation, except to cover up the random zit that never fails to make an appearance during that time of the month. The only topical skin care products that I use now are sunscreen, lip balm, bar soap, a facial cleanser, a hand and body lotion, and one or more botanical oils that I apply to my face and neck before bed in lieu of a night cream.

Fair to say, I do other things to help my skin look its best, such as getting plenty of sleep, drinking plenty of water, exercising several times a week, eating high-quality food, taking supplements, and minimizing stress. I wholeheartedly believe that topical products alone are not enough to maintain or achieve youthful skin. By the same token, adopting healthy habits in the absence of carefully chosen topical products is not without its own set of limitations. Therefore, if you want to look and feel young for most of your life, then it's crucial to approach this desire from all angles.

DIY Ageless Skin is meant to point you in the right direction with regard to the "topical" angle, although it does mention a few dietary and lifestyle considerations. When it comes to my routine and the nature of the products that I use, I prefer to keep things simple. This means using as few products as possible and choosing recipes that have as few ingredients as possible. (After more than about ten ingredients, the preparation becomes tedious, time-consuming, and expensive. Sometimes the best "recipes" have only one ingredient.) To that end, I seek out ingredients that offer multiple anti-aging benefits, as well as ingredients that are versatile in function. In other words, they can be used in a variety of products, such as lotions, lip balms, soaps, and more.

Keeping things simple saves time and money in the long run,* and it requires less storage space, which appeals to my minimalist tendencies. In addition, I believe that when it comes to anti-aging skin care and health in general, a preventive approach is the best. It's a lot more convenient to wait until you have a problem before looking for a solution, but the inconvenient truth is that many problems develop silently over time, and when they finally do surface, it can be difficult (and costly) to correct them.

---

*The challenge of doing more with less requires a budget for experimentation.

Although the anti-aging solutions mentioned in this book can improve one's appearance, there's no substitute for a lifetime of daily sunscreen application or other protective measures. In my opinion, if you're someone who's young enough to be wrinkle-free, then sunscreen is the best topical "anti-aging" product that money can buy. In Chapter 4, I discuss little-known facts about sunscreen and whether or not you should make your own.

2

THE STRUCTURE AND FUNCTION OF SKIN

Since the skin is a visual indicator of a person's overall health, it's beneficial to understand the basics of skin anatomy and physiology. Armed with this knowledge, you'll be able to better understand the aging process and why some products that you may be using are ineffective or counterproductive.

The skin is the largest organ of the human body, accounting for about 15% of one's total body weight. It protects the interior of the body from toxic substances, heat, excessive water loss, microorganisms, and ultraviolet radiation. Other major functions of the skin include vitamin D synthesis, temperature regulation, insulation, and the sensation of stimuli such as touch, pain, and warmth. The thickness of the skin varies across the body, but on average, it's approximately one millimeter (1 mm) thick and consists of two primary layers: the **epidermis** and the **dermis**. A third layer, the **hypodermis**, is often included in discussions of skin structure, but it's not really part of the skin. Another term for "skin" is "integument," and the skin itself is part of the integumentary system, which also includes the hair, nails, sebaceous glands, and sweat glands.

The Epidermis

The outermost layer of the integument is the epidermis. The epidermal layer itself is made up of five sublayers, listed below in order from top to bottom, with their alternate names in parentheses:

- Stratum corneum (horny layer)
- Stratum lucidum (clear layer)
- Stratum granulosum (granular layer)
- Stratum spinosum (spiny layer)
- Stratum basale (basal layer or stratum germinativum)

The **stratum basale** is the deepest layer of the epidermis. It contains a single layer of cells that separates the epidermis from the dermis. Five types of cells occupy the basal layer: stem cells, keratinocytes, melanocytes, Merkel cells, and Langerhans cells.

Stem cells are unspecialized cells that give rise to specialized cells through a process called **differentiation**. In the basal layer, epidermal stem cells rapidly divide to create cells that will become keratinocytes, whose "specialty" is to produce keratins. Keratins (sometimes collectively called "keratin") are proteins that help give the skin strength and make it resistant to environmental toxins and physical stress. Similarly, melanocyte stem cells give rise to melanocytes, whose function is to produce and store melanin, the pigment that gives the skin its color and photoprotection. When skin gets tanned upon exposure to ultraviolet (UV) light from the sun or a tanning bed, what's happening is that melanocytes are transferring pigment granules called melanosomes into the keratinocytes. The melanosomes then gather around the nucleus of the keratinocyte to shield the cell's DNA from the harmful UV rays. People with naturally darker skin tones have more melanin and are less prone to sun damage than fair-skinned people.

In addition to keratinocytes and melanocytes, the basal layer is home to Merkel cells and Langerhans cells. Merkel cells, or tactile cells, are few in number and sensitive to touch. When something touches your skin, they release chemicals that stimulate sensory nerve endings, which in turn let the brain know that you were touched in that area. Langerhans cells are also few in number relative to keratinocytes, and their function is to detect pathogens and alert the immune system to respond accordingly. Although Langerhans cells are present in all layers of the epidermis, they're most prevalent in the stratum spinosum.

The **stratum spinosum** consists of several layers of keratinocytes. The cells that were made in the stratum basale are pushed into this layer, where they begin to develop into specialized, non-dividing keratinocytes. Some of the cells in the stratum basale are still dividing, though. Once mature, they'll start producing keratin.

In the **stratum granulosum**, there are three to five layers of keratinocytes. This is the first layer of keratinization, in which the keratinocytes fill up with keratin. Consequently, each cell's nucleus and organelles disintegrate. A fully keratinized cell is biologically dead but structurally sound. The keratinization process, however, is incomplete until the cells continue moving upward into the stratum lucidum and the stratum corneum.

The **stratum lucidum** has two to three layers of keratinocytes and is found only in areas of thick skin, such as the palms of hands and the soles of feet. The purpose of the stratum lucidum is to reduce friction between the stratum granulosum and the stratum corneum.

The **stratum corneum** is the most superficial layer of the epidermis and is the part of skin that we can see. It's sometimes called the "horny layer" because of the way it looks under the powerful magnification of an electron microscope. This region is made up of 20 to 30 layers of dead, flattened, interlocking keratinized cells that have no nucleus and are tightly packed together. Even though these cells have lost their nuclei and organelles, they still contain many types of molecules—keratin, lipids, and ceramides—that are essential to the skin's role as a protective barrier.

The vast majority of cells within the epidermis are keratinocytes. The deepest three layers (stratum basale, spinosum, and granulosum) of the epidermis contain living keratinocytes, while the top two layers (stratum lucidum and corneum) contain dead keratinocytes that are eventually shed and replaced by the newer cells beneath them. During their migration from the stratum basale to the stratum corneum, keratinocytes undergo various structural changes, and they remain in the stratum corneum until they are shed. This process of skin regeneration, or skin renewal, takes about 30 days but varies with age. In the elderly, it may take as many as 50 days for the cell migration and shedding to occur, which is one reason why wounds take longer to heal as we get older. When a skin care product is said to have "regenerative properties," that means that one or more of its ingredients can speed up the renewal process. Many botanical oils are prized for their regenerative abilities. When it comes to wrinkles, however, these oils are most effective as a preventive measure, rather than a corrective one. (Incidentally, they can also be used to prevent the formation of stretch marks during pregnancy or rapid muscle building.) Although wrinkles are visible in the epidermis, they're actually formed in the dermis. Therefore, any wrinkle treatment will be ineffective unless the active ingredients can penetrate the five sublayers of the epidermis to reach the dermis, where they're needed most.

The Dermis

The dermis connects the epidermis to the rest of the body and consists of two sublayers: the papillary layer and the reticular layer. The upper, papillary region contains a chaotic arrangement of thin fibers made of **collagen**, a protein that gives the skin its strength and firmness. Below this mass of collagen is the reticular region, consisting of another layer of collagen. However, the collagen fibers here are thicker and usually run in a direction that is parallel to the surface of the skin. The fibers are all interconnected, thus forming a network. (The reticular layer gets its name from "reticulum," the Latin word for "network.") This networked structure has immense tensile strength and holds the skin tissue together like glue.

In addition to collagen, the dermis contains another type of protein called **elastin**, whose function is to return many tissues in the body to their original shape after being stretched or contracted. As its name implies, elastin is responsible for the skin's elasticity, or ability to resume its normal form after being poked or pinched. Both collagen and elastin are made in the dermis by specialized cells called fibroblasts. Healthy fibroblasts are crucial for healthy skin.

Also present in the dermis are blood vessels, lymph vessels, hair follicles, sweat glands, sebaceous glands, and specialized nerve cells. The blood vessels provide nourishment and waste removal for both dermal and epidermal cells, while the lymph vessels act as reservoirs for plasma and other substances, including cells that have leaked from the vascular system. They also transport lymph fluid back from the tissues to the circulatory system. Without functioning lymph vessels, lymph cannot be effectively drained, and edema (swelling due to the abnormal accumulation of fluid) typically results.

The sweat glands create a watery, salty fluid known as sweat or perspiration, and the sebaceous glands produce an oily or waxy substance called **sebum**. The purpose of sebum is to lubricate and waterproof the skin and hair. Sebaceous glands are found on all parts of the skin except the palms of hands and soles of feet. They're most prevalent in the face and scalp, and overactive sebaceous glands in either of these areas can lead to undesirable conditions, such as acne, oily skin, or dandruff. Underactive sebaceous glands produce too little oil, leading to dry skin. The body's continuous secretion of both sweat and sebum forms a thin, slightly acidic film on the surface of the epidermis that holds moisture in and acts as a barrier to microbes and other potential contaminants. This film is the **acid mantle**.

Unfortunately, many commercial "soaps" and shampoos are actually detergents that strip away the acid mantle, causing dryness and a subsequent need for a moisturizer (or a conditioner in the case of shampoo). By contrast, bar soap that is handcrafted from vegetable oils and lye rarely leads to dry, itchy skin. In fact, many people who switch to handmade soap are often surprised at how much it improves their quality of life.[1] In some cases, however, a person's age or diet, or the climate in which he or she lives, may be contributing to dry skin, so using a moisturizer of some kind is still necessary.

Skin produces less sebum as we age, and chronic nutrient insufficiencies often take their toll on the integumentary system. For example, not getting enough essential fatty acids (EFAs) can cause the skin and hair to become dry. EFAs must be obtained through the diet because our bodies cannot make them. Increasing one's intake of EFAs can make the skin and hair feel soft and look more youthful. Some botanical oils are rich sources of EFAs and can be used for culinary and/or beauty purposes. Applying the oils directly to the skin and hair can help to reduce water loss and serve as a substitute for sebum. This works particularly well when using oils that have a similar chemical composition to sebum.

While dry skin can make existing lines and wrinkles appear more prominent, it's important to understand that wrinkles are not actually caused by dry skin. They're formed in the dermis, where it's always moist. Oxidative stress caused by UV radiation and smoking is the leading cause of wrinkles. Facial expressions that result in skin folding are another cause of wrinkling, and such wrinkles can even be seen in children and young adults. Genetics and the natural aging process contribute to wrinkling as well, but in the latter case, there are certain dietary and lifestyle changes that you can make to look and feel younger (and to possibly reverse medical conditions that may be wreaking havoc on your life, but I digress).

The Hypodermis

Many of the glands and cells present in the dermis are also found in the hypodermis, the region between the dermis and muscle. It mainly consists of loose connective tissue, with a vast quantity of adipose (fat) cells. At the base of the hypodermis and throughout the hypodermis are a series of veins, arteries, and lymph channels, which collectively regulate blood flow. There are also nerves to receive touch sensations.

Technically, the hypodermis is not part of the integument, but it's worth mentioning because of its relevance to the aging process. As we get older, the amount of fat in the hypodermis decreases, causing the skin to sag and wrinkles to look more defined. People of any age can experience sagging skin if they have lost a lot of weight during a relatively short period of time. Therefore, if you're planning to lose weight, it's best to avoid methods that can result in rapid weight loss, such as low-carb diets or severe caloric restriction.

The body interprets rapid weight loss as trauma and responds by shutting down certain "unnecessary activities," if you will, not the least of which is hair growth. The hair on your head is not required for survival, so the body can afford to lose it in times of stress. A temporary, non-genetic form of hair loss called **telogen effluvium** may occur about three months after experiencing some kind of trauma. Most often, it's emotional or psychological trauma, but it could be physical trauma as well, such as surgery.

Normally, we lose about 100 hairs a day, but in telogen effluvium, several hundred hairs may be lost in one day, leaving the victim clueless as to what's going on, since whatever caused the hair loss happened months ago and is probably long forgotten. In chronically traumatic situations, shedding will continue until its root cause is eliminated. Following the period of excessive shedding, it usually takes a few more months for new hair to start growing back. Hair loss is not something that many people associate with weight loss, but it does happen. Bariatric surgery and very low caloric intake are common causes of the type of hair loss that may accompany rapid weight loss. If you plan to make any radical changes to your body, diet, or lifestyle, it may be wise to execute them slowly over time if the circumstances will allow it. Patience really is a virtue.

3

WHAT HAPPENS TO THE SKIN AS WE AGE?

Everyone knows that as we get older, our skin develops fine lines and wrinkles. But how exactly does this happen, and is there anything you can do about it before or after the fact? This chapter is about the structural changes that occur in the skin during the aging process, while later chapters cover what steps you can take to mitigate the effects of those changes.

Intrinsic vs. Extrinsic Aging

The aging of the skin and other parts of the integumentary system can be described as intrinsic or extrinsic. **Intrinsic aging**, or chronological aging, is caused by internal physiological factors that normally change with the passing of time, whereas **extrinsic aging** is caused by external factors, such as air pollution, sun exposure, and lifestyle choices. Although extrinsic aging may occur for a variety of reasons, it's largely the result of damage caused by UV radiation. As such, it's commonly referred to as **photoaging**.

Aging affects the skin and internal organs in a similar way. Like keratinocytes, the majority of other types of cells also have life cycles. They gradually reach **senescence**, meaning that they remain viable but incapable of reproducing. Over time, these natural changes lead to faulty responses to environmental factors, which in turn lead to cell death. Changes also occur in part due to cumulative damage from oxidative stress or the continuous formation of **reactive oxygen species** (ROS). Despite the body's strong antioxidant defense system, damage caused by ROS affects cell membranes, enzymes, and DNA. Eventually, other molecules and hormones decline as well, resulting in an aging body and aging skin.

The Aging Epidermis

There are four major distinctions between young and aged skin: epidermal thinning, wrinkles, a flattened dermal-epidermal junction (DEJ), and collagen fragmentation. The aging epidermis is characterized by a thinner appearance and a slower cell turnover rate. As discussed in the previous chapter, the epidermis forms a barrier against the environment and transepidermal water loss. Specialized epidermal cells called keratinocytes divide and make their way from the base of the epidermis to the surface, where they are shed and then replaced by newer cells.

With aged skin, the cell turnover and renewal process slows down, and the epidermis becomes impaired. The impairment results in dehydration, delayed wound healing, and the appearance of fine lines. Less effective **desquamation** (the normal, non-pathologic shedding of keratinocytes in the stratum corneum) results in excess stratum corneum layers that make the skin look dull. In addition, the amount of lipids produced by our skin decreases as we age. Lipids are crucial for maintaining the skin's protective function and for preventing the excessive loss of water and electrolytes. There's also a decreased number of melanocytes and Langerhans cells within the aging epidermis. The reduction in melanocytes produces the mottled pigmentation that's common in elderly skin, which appears more prominent in sun-exposed areas like the face and hands.

The Aging Dermis and Hypodermis

As we age, the dermis loses volume, and there's less nutrient transfer due to a reduction in the number of blood vessels. There's also reduced sensory innervation of nerves into the skin, which may explain why certain sensations become harder to perceive with age. Both the dermis and hypodermis become atrophied, with a reduction in collagen, glycosaminoglycans (GAGs), and adipose tissue. Collagen is an important component of the DEJ, and it forms a highly cross-linked network that is necessary for mechanical stability and support. GAGs are important molecules in the dermis for consolidating collagen fibers and assisting with skin hydration. Reduced collagen and GAGs with age or sun exposure can weaken the mechanical stability of the skin and allow the formation of a wrinkle. These reductions give rise to skin that is less elastic. Skin appendages are also affected by aging in that there are fewer sweat glands, and less sebum is produced. Terminal hairs turn to vellus hairs, and the loss of melanocytes in hair bulbs causes the hair to turn gray.

Photoaging

UV radiation is the largest contributor to extrinsic aging, especially in premature skin aging. There are two types of UV rays that cause skin damage: UVA and UVB. UVB rays alter skin structure, mainly at the level of the epidermis, where most of them are absorbed. Here, UVB can damage DNA in melanocytes and keratinocytes, and it can also cause sunburns. UVA rays penetrate more deeply into the dermis and play an important role in the pathology of photoaging. UVA causes oxidative stress, mainly by the production of ROS. In photoaged skin, collagen fibrils (fine collagen fibers) are disorganized, and UV radiation increases the production of collagen-degrading enzymes, such as the matrix metalloproteinases (MMPs).

MMPs are a collection of enzymes that degrade or break down the extracellular matrix in the dermis. Each MMP is a family of enzymes responsible for breaking down a specific component of the matrix. Collagenase, elastase, and hyaluronidase break down collagen, elastin, and hyaluronic acid, respectively. The remodeling of connective tissue by MMPs is an important process in aging and wound healing, and the MMPs are normally called to action only when needed. However, inflammation and UV radiation will also call them into action, and this can result in disorganized and clumped collagen, which is characteristic of photoaged skin. Moreover, the natural inhibitors of MMPs in skin diminish with age, resulting in more MMP action and less collagen.

Many skin cells, including immune cells (Langerhans cells), pigment cells (melanocytes), and signaling molecules that trigger inflammation, are altered by UV radiation. The culmination of DNA damage from UV rays is skin cancer, which is prevalent in certain climates, especially in people with lighter skin. Sunscreen, protective clothing, and minimal sun exposure are the mainstays in the prevention of photoaging.

What Exactly Is a Wrinkle?

Wrinkles are folds of the skin, more frequently seen on the face and hands because these areas get the most sun exposure during a person's lifetime. (Sun damage is cumulative and begins the day you're born.) Wrinkle formation is the result of numerous structural changes in the dermis and epidermis that are caused by both intrinsic and extrinsic factors. As we age, our bodies produce less collagen and elastin, the proteins responsible for our skin's strength and elasticity. Decreased production of these important fibers, in combination with their abnormal formation as a result of UV damage, weakens the skin and leads to wrinkles and sagging. Other factors, such as smoking, alcoholism, pollution, diet, and stress, diminish the body's ability to maintain youthful, healthy looking skin.

The skin is particularly susceptible to ROS or oxidative damage. ROS, also referred to as **free radicals**, can cause lipid peroxidation, which is damaging to cell membranes. This can result in premature aging, skin cancer, and even cell death. Antioxidants are the body's natural defense against oxidative stress. They include vitamins C and E, minerals, enzymes like superoxide dismutase (SOD) and catalase, and naturally occurring proteins that are found in our bodies or obtained through our diet. When these defenses become overwhelmed, free radicals will cause damage. On the skin, this translates to wrinkles, hyperpigmentation, and inflammation.

Free radicals (atoms, molecules, or ions with an unpaired electron) are generated during many biochemical reactions in the body. They're highly reactive toward other molecules or among themselves because having an unpaired electron is chemically unstable. A chemical bond results from a shared pair of electrons between two adjacent atoms in a molecule, and a missing electron causes the free radical to "seek out" another atom or molecule with which to bond. Sometimes this is good, and sometimes it's not. In the skin, free radicals generated by a process called **glycation** attack collagen and elastin fibers, causing them to become malformed. When they're in that state, they can't be broken down properly by MMPs. Consequently, the skin becomes stiff and takes on a yellowish-brown color.

Glycation also generates molecules referred to as **advanced glycation end products** (AGEs). These were first identified in cooked food as end products from the non-enzymatic reaction between sugars and proteins. In the kitchen, you can observe glycation in action when browning meat or toasting bread. In humans, glycation occurs slowly and affects aging, as well as several different diseases. As we age, there's a higher risk of glycation-induced damage to the skin. Therefore, it's important to prevent the action of AGEs and to prevent future oxidative damage from free radicals. These biochemical reactions, combined with the natural progression of biological aging, are what bring about fine lines, wrinkles, pigmentation, texture changes, and loss of tensile strength.

What Happens to Your Skin Through Each Decade of Life?

In your twenties, the skin is supple and has great collagen support. Whatever skin damage you may have is probably not yet visible, and cell turnover is about 14-25 days. In your thirties, you might start noticing fine lines and wrinkles, especially around the mouth and eyes. You may notice discoloration and uneven skin tone. Your skin may be thinner as a result of some collagen loss, and cell turnover begins to slow down to about 30 days, making your complexion a little dull.

In your forties, cumulative sun damage appears in the form of blotchiness, red spots, and even ruddiness. You lose more collagen and elastin, and the skin retains less moisture. Cell turnover is about 40 days. In your fifties and beyond, there's more dryness and loss of elasticity. Expression lines no longer disappear after you stop laughing or smiling. Pores are more visible, especially in the nose and cheeks. Spider veins and hyperpigmentation may now be visible, along with pre-cancerous spots from sun damage, such as actinic keratosis. In women, menopause can result in dryness, decreased elasticity, and loss of dermal volume. Cell turnover can take at least 50 days.

Can Wrinkles Be Prevented or "Erased"?

If you're young and take excellent care of your skin through each phase of your life, then you can bank on always looking several years younger than you really are, assuming that you take excellent care of your mind and body as well. In the long run, makeup and skin care products are no match for chronic stress, depression, sleep deprivation, substance abuse, or poor nutrition. If, on the other hand, you're getting up in years, then you'll be pleased to know that by making certain changes to the way you care for your skin and overall health, you may be able to prevent further skin damage and, in some cases, reverse it—all without having to consult with a dermatologist or subject yourself to costly, painful, or invasive procedures.

Intrinsic aging is inevitable, whereas extrinsic aging can result from factors that are within your control. Having said that, it's possible to manipulate some aspects of your physiology to delay or reverse aging at the cellular level, thereby making yourself look and feel much younger. If you exercise patience (there's that word again) and stay committed to your regimen, you could very well experience the vigor of your twenties again, even if you're in your fifties now. By focusing on repair strategies, you can minimize or halt the activity of overactive MMPs, AGEs, and destructive ROS. You can also help rebuild the dermal matrix to support the skin, as well as prevent accelerated aging with effective sun protection in conjunction with antioxidants, vitamins, and minerals.

4
SUNSCREEN AND PHOTOAGING

Wearing sunscreen is critical to avoiding premature skin aging. This is widely known, and yet so many people are reluctant to use it for whatever reason:

- "I'm only going to the store and back."
- "It's cloudy."
- "I work inside all day."
- "It's not summer yet."
- "That stuff is too greasy."
- "I don't want to smell like I'm going to the beach unless I *am* going to the beach."

While it's understandable to be turned off by the texture and fragrance of typical sunscreens, the other reasons for not using it are due to misconceptions about UV radiation and the harm that it can do over time. Sun protection is not just about avoiding sunburns. It's also about preventing wrinkles, age spots, and skin cancer. Since UV-related skin damage is cumulative, quick outings "to the store and back" (or having a desk job) will eventually catch up with you if you're not diligent about using sunscreen. Women tend to be mindful of this fact, but they only seem to care about their faces, not their necks, hands, and other areas of exposed skin. It's not uncommon to see a middle-aged woman with a young-ish face and a neck that looks much older. This chapter covers important information about UV radiation, sun protection, and whether you should make your own sunscreen or put your faith in Coppertone®.

UVA vs. UVB Radiation

There are two types of UV radiation that we need to be aware of for the purposes of preventing skin damage: ultraviolet A (UVA) and ultraviolet B (UVB). UVB light is responsible for causing reddening and sunburn. UVA light doesn't cause burning, but it does travel deep into the dermis, where it can harm living skin cells (the cells on the surface of the skin are dead). UVA light also causes the skin to darken and is the predominant type of UV ray used in tanning beds. This darkening process is called **melanogenesis**, and it's the skin's way of protecting itself from cellular DNA damage by increasing the production of melanin, the pigment that gives skin its color.

Both UVA and UVB rays contribute to skin cancer and premature aging. The best way to protect your skin from harmful UV radiation is to use sunscreen on a daily basis, even if you spend most of your time indoors. Glass doesn't protect you from all UV radiation; it blocks only UVB radiation. Another distinction between UVA and UVB radiation is that UVA rays are equally intense throughout the year during all daylight hours, whereas UVB rays are most intense during the summer, at high altitudes, and between the hours of 10:00 a.m. and 2:00 p.m. Also keep in mind that ultraviolet A and B rays pass through the clouds, so it's important to wear sunscreen on gray days, too.

Sun Protection Factor (SPF)

The sun protection factor (SPF) applies only to UVB radiation and has no relevance to UVA radiation. SPF is a measure of how long it will take, in theory, for your skin to burn. For example, if you normally burn after being in the sun for 20 minutes without sunscreen, then a product with SPF 15 would allow you to be in the sun for 15 times your burn time. In this case, that would be 300 minutes (five hours). Burn times vary from one person to the next, so the SPF value should be used only as a guide.

SPF values may also be thought of in terms of the percentage of UVB light that gets filtered. While no sunscreen has the ability to protect you from 100% of UV radiation, most sunscreens filter out the vast majority of incoming UVB rays. An SPF 15 product filters out approximately 93% of UVB rays, and an SPF 30 product filters out approximately 97% of UVB rays. Using an SPF 50 sunscreen results in only a 1% increase in filtering ability relative to an SPF 30 sunscreen.

Because SPF values above 30 don't offer what scientists consider to be "significant" gains in sun protection, it's illegal in some countries to sell sunscreen products that are above SPF 30. Despite what the "science" tells us, some consumers find that they burn too easily with SPF 30 sunscreens and opt for sunscreens with an SPF of 50 or higher. Fair to say, some people who have gotten a sunburn while using sunscreen may have been guilty of not following the directions on the label, but there are others who did everything right and still got burned, myself included.

As with all products that are meant for the skin, only you can be the judge of what "works" or not, but here's something to consider: the SPF number on a product's label is often higher than the actual SPF. The reason is that a product's SPF value is determined in a laboratory setting, where a specific and uniform density of sunscreen is applied and then tested. In the real world, there is less control over how the product is used. The typical consumer will apply the sunscreen to his or her skin at about half of the lab-validated density or even less, so the actual SPF will be lower than what it says on the label. Interestingly, it has been shown that high-SPF sunscreens can compensate for under-application of lower-SPF sunscreens.[2]

Broad Spectrum Sunscreen

The **ultraviolet spectrum** is a subset of the **electromagnetic spectrum**, which includes the entire range of electromagnetic radiation.[3] UVA light ranges from 320 nanometers (nm) to 400 nm, and UVB light ranges from 290-320 nm. There's also UVC light (200-290 nm), but it gets absorbed by the atmosphere and ozone layer before it can reach the surface of the earth. Therefore, it's not considered to be a threat to skin health. In order to protect yourself against both UVA and UVB radiation, it's important to use a sunscreen product that offers so-called "broad spectrum" protection. Not all "SPF" products meet this criterion, so be sure to check the label. A lack of broad spectrum protection is especially common with moisturizers.

Inorganic vs. Organic Sunscreens

In the context of chemistry, "organic" means that the substance in question contains carbon. Organic molecules are typically composed of carbon, hydrogen, nitrogen, and oxygen atoms. By contrast, "inorganic" molecules do not contain any carbon, although they may contain hydrogen, nitrogen, oxygen, or other atoms.

When it comes to sunscreen, you have a choice between organic and inorganic products. The active ingredients of organic sunscreens are synthetic compounds that do not occur in nature, while the active ingredients of inorganic sunscreens are natural minerals that, for logistical reasons, are produced synthetically on an industrial scale. Several organic compounds have sunscreen activity, but only two inorganic compounds are approved for use as sunscreens: zinc oxide (ZnO) and titanium dioxide (TiO_2). Zinc oxide offers the most powerful broad-spectrum protection of all sunscreen active ingredients, inorganic or otherwise.[4] Titanium dioxide also has the ability to protect against both UVA and UVB rays, but it's not as effective as zinc oxide in the UVA range.

Organic and inorganic sunscreens are sometimes referred to as "chemical" or "physical" sunscreens, respectively. Of course, they're both chemicals, but the concept behind these terms has to do with how they protect the skin against UV damage. Organic sunscreens are absorbed into the skin and offer protection by absorbing UV radiation. When UV rays are absorbed, these active ingredients chemically degrade. Once they're degraded, they no longer offer any UV protection, and this is why organic sunscreens must be reapplied every two hours (or more often if you'll be swimming or sweating). The initial application should also be done at least 15 minutes before sun exposure to give the sunscreen time to become absorbed.

Instead of being absorbed into the skin and chemically reacting upon exposure to UV light, inorganic sunscreens sit on top of the skin, thus forming a physical barrier between you and the sun. While both zinc and titanium dioxides do absorb UV radiation to a certain extent, they're chemically inert and don't face the degradation problem of organic sunscreens. They do, however, have a fatal flaw: if you brush up against something or wipe your skin for some other reason, the inorganic sunscreen will rub off and need to be reapplied. You'll know when it happens because zinc and titanium dioxides leave a white mark on anything they touch. This is a drawback to using a mineral-based sunscreen, but should you happen to get it on your clothes, rest assured that the white marks are not stains and that they'll come out in the wash. Other affected surfaces can be wiped clean with a damp cloth.

Mineral sunscreens also tend to leave a white cast on the skin, but that has a lot to do with the particle size of the mineral. When it comes to inorganic sunscreen, you have a choice between "nano" (as in "nanoparticles" and "nanotechnology") and "non-nano" products. Some manufacturers use nanoparticles of zinc oxide because they have more favorable cosmetic properties, namely that they "go on clear" instead of making the skin look ghostly white. Other manufacturers claim that nanoparticles of zinc oxide are capable of penetrating the skin and getting absorbed into the bloodstream, so they market their products as "non-nano." Unfortunately, the larger particle size is not as effective in terms of UV protection, due to the decrease in particle concentration.[5] In other words, larger particles cannot be packed together as tightly as smaller particles, and the result is more space between the particles. Empty space is unprotected space.

Should You Make Your Own Sunscreen?

People who make their own sunscreen tend to be motivated by wanting to use only ingredients that are both natural and non-toxic, which, in their opinion, leaves zinc oxide and titanium dioxide as the only options. Their concern with organic sunscreens is two-fold: they're potential endocrine disruptors, and some of them produce free radicals when exposed to sunlight. Free radicals cause damage to the skin that results in cancer and premature aging, two problems that sunscreens are meant to avoid. The safety of inorganic sunscreens is equally controversial, as some people argue that nanoparticles of zinc and titanium dioxide can penetrate the skin and enter the bloodstream, while others have concluded that it doesn't happen. After much research, I still haven't formed an opinion on the safety of nano-sized mineral oxides over organic sunscreens. I do, however, prefer the "experience" of using mineral sunscreens because I don't normally wear foundation, and inorganic products offer the light coverage that I'm looking for without making my face look like it was painted white.

Now let's assume for a moment that inorganic sunscreens are safer than organic sunscreens. If you choose to make your own product based on that assumption, then you still face the challenges of determining efficacy and coming up with a formulation that results in a uniform consistency so that the product isn't lumpy like tapioca pudding. Lumpiness is an issue because zinc and titanium dioxides aren't soluble in water or oil. Therefore, they must be suspended or dispersed in your lotion/cream base. A lack of uniform particle density can result in areas of uneven coverage and sun protection when applied to the skin.

Furthermore, the only way to know the SPF of the product is to have it tested by a lab, and that costs hundreds of dollars per test.

Making a mineral-based sunscreen that contains natural products exclusively is not as easy as it may seem from reading various DIY skin care blogs. Although I have made my own, and it works in the sense that I haven't gotten sunburned, nor have I noticed any melanogenesis going on, I have yet to come up with a recipe that I'm truly happy with. The variations that I've tried so far are all too greasy, even when using a "matte" oil such as red raspberry seed oil. (Using less oil would result in a product that doesn't spread easily on the skin.)

I've gone back to using a commercial sunscreen for the time being, and fortunately, there are several inorganic sunscreens on the market to choose from. If you want to try them yourself, you may have to order them online because big-box stores and pharmacies tend to stock their shelves with organic sunscreens only, especially during the "off season" (but you know better than to wait for summer). I've listed a few inorganic sun protection products on my website that you may be interested in. If you live near any specialty health food stores, that might be another option for purchasing them.

5

SHOULD YOU MAKE YOUR OWN VITAMIN C SERUM?

Vitamin C serums are all the rage in the anti-aging skin care industry because topical use of vitamin C has been shown to promote collagen synthesis[6-7] and mitigate photodamage caused by ROS.[8-10] Although oral supplementation with vitamin C (also known as L-ascorbic acid or ascorbic acid) may benefit one's overall health, topical formulations are often preferred for addressing skin problems. Since vitamin C is needed for a host of functions within the body, certain biochemical mechanisms ration the quantity of vitamin C delivered to the skin after oral ingestion. Therefore, increasing one's intake of vitamin C doesn't always correspond to an increase in vitamin C in the skin. When vitamin C is applied topically, the regulatory mechanisms are bypassed, and therapeutic doses can reach the living cells of the epidermis and dermis.

Despite this good news, L-ascorbic acid has a few issues. It's a notoriously unstable, water-soluble compound that doesn't penetrate the skin easily, which makes sense when you consider the structure of the epidermis. The stratum corneum (the topmost layer of skin) is made up of dead, keratinized cells embedded in an extracellular lipid matrix.[11-12] This layer of the epidermis is often described as having a "brick and mortar" type of structure where the keratinocytes are the bricks, and the lipids are the mortar. In order for L-ascorbic acid to get past this brick wall, it must be in its free form (i.e., un-ionized), and the pH of the solution must be no higher than 3.5. Maximal skin penetration occurs at a pH of 2.0 (very acidic) and an L-ascorbic acid concentration of 20%.[13] Unfortunately, the high acidity causes stinging and irritation when aqueous L-ascorbic acid is applied to the skin. Using a low concentration can alleviate this problem, but still not everyone's skin can tolerate it, and lower concentrations may not achieve the desired results. L-ascorbic acid is exfoliating as well, and exfoliating too frequently can damage your skin.

To combat these problems, some cosmetic formulators have found ways to make vitamin C serums a bit more stable and less irritating, while others have opted to forego L-ascorbic acid in favor of its many derivatives. In chemistry, a derivative is a compound that is derived from a similar compound by some chemical or physical process. Vitamin C derivatives that are commonly used in skin care products are: ascorbyl palmitate, tetrahexyldecyl ascorbate (also known as ascorbyl tetra-isopalmitate), sodium ascorbyl phosphate, and magnesium ascorbyl phosphate. The advantages of using vitamin C derivatives are greater chemical stability, little or no skin irritation, and no exfoliating action. These derivatives, however, are not infallible. While they're less prone to oxidation than L-ascorbic acid, they're not immune to it. Furthermore, the concentrations of vitamin C derivatives used in many products may be adequate for antioxidant functionality but insufficient for collagen synthesis.

Before deciding to make a DIY vitamin C serum, please take into account the following additional considerations.

1) How will you formulate your serum to maximize stability, absorption, and effectiveness while minimizing skin irritation and toxicity?

L-ascorbic acid is sensitive to light, heat, air, and humidity. In order to get the most benefit out of a DIY vitamin C serum, it should be made in small batches and kept refrigerated in an airtight, dark glass bottle. Since it oxidizes quickly, it should be used within a few days. Ideally, your serum should be used immediately after making it, especially if you choose not to add any stabilizing agents, such as vitamin E and/or ferulic acid.[14] If you do wish to stabilize the vitamin C, then you'll be faced with a solubility challenge because L-ascorbic acid is water-soluble, whereas vitamin E and ferulic acid are not. Choosing to model your L-ascorbic acid serum after a commercial one may also prove to be difficult because you won't know the concentrations of all ingredients, nor the exact method of preparation. Simply mixing all of the ingredients together at once is not always how such products are made. You'll also need to control the pH of your serum to ensure that the L-ascorbic acid will be able to penetrate the skin.

If you're leaning toward using a vitamin C derivative to deal with the inherent problems of L-ascorbic acid, then it's important to be aware that its derivatives have problems, too. Because L-ascorbic acid is the only biologically active form of vitamin C, the body must be able to convert the vitamin C derivative into L-ascorbic acid in order for it to be effective. Ascorbyl palmitate in particular may penetrate the skin better than L-ascorbic acid because it's fat-soluble, but its conversion to the active form of vitamin C is "inefficient,"[15-16] and the amount of ascorbyl palmitate required to achieve physiologic levels of L-ascorbic acid may be toxic.[17]

In addition to being aware of an ingredient's potential toxicity, it's also important to know the correct amount of derivative to use in order to achieve the results that you want. For example, in an experiment that tested the abilities of magnesium ascorbyl phosphate (MAP) and sodium ascorbyl phosphate (SAP) to stimulate collagen synthesis relative to L-ascorbic acid, it was found that MAP was equivalent to ascorbic acid, while SAP "required at least a tenfold greater concentration to produce the same effect as ascorbic acid."[18] Regardless of whether you use L-ascorbic acid or one of its derivatives, don't underestimate the the value of due diligence. Research each ingredient thoroughly in terms of solubility, stability, absorption, toxicity, effective concentrations, and side effects.

2) While making your own products can be empowering, it's important to be mindful of unintended consequences.

For example, collagen and elastin work together to maintain the structural integrity of the skin, but even though topical vitamin C can promote collagen synthesis, it appears to do so at the expense of elastin.[19]

This could be good or bad, depending on the current condition of your skin. Since elastin accumulates abnormally in photoaged skin, vitamin C might help prevent this from occurring to an appreciable extent. It may, however, interfere with normal elastin production in healthy, non-photoaged skin. If your goal is to heal photodamage, then topical ascorbic acid might be your ticket, but if your goal is to prevent wrinkles, then this approach might be counterproductive until you reach a certain age. (Vitamin C levels in the skin decline with age.)[20-22]

3) Topical vitamin C can help protect against oxidative damage, but vitamin C alone is not enough.

The body's innate ability to defend itself against ROS relies on the synergistic cooperation of multiple antioxidants. This is in part due to the medium in which the oxidative stress occurs. The water-soluble vitamin C protects the aqueous parts of the skin, such as tissues and cellular fluids, while the fat-soluble vitamin E protects the lipid membranes of skin cells.[23] Vitamin C also has the ability to regenerate vitamin E, and the combination of topical vitamins C and E has been shown to be more effective than vitamin C alone in terms of photoprotection.[24] In addition, many fruits and vegetables contain a variety of antioxidants that can endogenously protect your skin from sun damage[25] (but diet alone shouldn't be relied upon because many factors affect the body's ability to absorb and use nutrients).

With regard to dietary antioxidants, it's worth mentioning that for all of the hype surrounding them, their antioxidant strength is actually weak in comparison to **glutathione**, the most powerful and abundant antioxidant in the human body. A deficiency of glutathione leads to oxidative stress,[26] a well-known cause of aging. Dr. Marcus L. Gitterle, author of *Growing Young*, has the following to say about the antioxidants that we obtain from so-called healthy diets: "What you need to know about free radicals is that our main defense against them is in the form of a built-in paramilitary force that makes the smoothie, green tea and multivitamin combo look like a bunch of rank amateurs. Comparing it to those garden variety antioxidants would be like sending the neighborhood watch team to Iraq to help out." He goes on to discuss the importance of glutathione's roles in the body and what you can do to raise your glutathione level. (Taking a glutathione supplement is not the answer because the glutathione would be broken down during digestion, so it would never reach the cells where it's needed.)

4) In terms of boosting collagen synthesis, ascorbic acid doesn't work for everybody.

In a study[7] involving 10 postmenopausal women from ages 50 to 60, it was discovered that the topical L-ascorbic acid treatment had no significant effect on collagen synthesis in the participants with the highest dietary intakes of vitamin C, and that their response to the treatment was unrelated to the amount of photodamage. The researchers also state that "the functional activity of the dermal cells is not maximal in postmenopausal women and can be increased," which implies that one's biologic age doesn't have to match one's chronologic age. *You can't stop the passing of time, but you can make your body perform like a younger version of itself.* This is a major theme in holistic anti-aging skin care and one that I hope you will adopt if you haven't already. If you're interested in learning how to slow or reverse aging at the cellular level, then pick up a copy of *Growing Young: A Doctor's Guide to the NEW Anti-Aging.*

The Bottom Line

Creating a vitamin C serum that serves its intended purpose without leading to undesirable consequences is far from trivial. Both endogenous photoprotection and collagen synthesis are complex biological processes involving several nutrients, not just vitamin C. Minimizing stress is also crucial because cortisol, the "stress hormone," inhibits collagen production. Therefore, it stands to reason that supporting the skin from the inside out through diet, supplements, and a healthy lifestyle is an invaluable key to healing damage and maintaining a more youthful appearance. On the other hand, "DIY" is about having the freedom to make personal choices about what you put on your skin (and into your body), so if you believe that topical vitamin C is appropriate for your needs, then give it a try. The purpose of this chapter is merely to give you some points to think about before buying a bottle of L-ascorbic acid.

6

BOTANICAL OILS: STABLE AND EFFECTIVE ALTERNATIVES TO TOPICAL VITAMIN C

The UV-induced destruction of collagen by matrix metalloproteinases leads to wrinkles and is the main contributor to extrinsic aging.[27] Ultraviolet radiation can also cause dark spots (hyperpigmentation) to appear on the skin of people with a long history of unprotected sun exposure. Both of these issues, as well as transepidermal water loss, can be addressed by using a topical vitamin C serum, but whether you buy a serum or make your own, there's no escaping the inherent problems of L-ascorbic acid and its derivatives. If you had high hopes for vitamin C serums before reading this book, then don't worry, all is not lost. You'll be pleased to know that the anti-aging benefits of topical vitamin C can be achieved through other means. If you share my skin care philosophy and would prefer to use as few products as possible to get the job done at a reasonable cost, then botanical oils deserve your consideration. Not only do they tend to be a lot more chemically stable than topical L-ascorbic acid, they're also more versatile in terms of their health benefits. Some of the oils are edible and can be incorporated into your diet as a source of antioxidants, essential fatty acids (vitamin F), and vitamins A, D, E, and K.

The anti-aging effects of botanical oils are in part due to their high essential fatty acid (EFA) content. EFAs are necessary for the proper functioning of the nervous, circulatory, and immune systems, as well as the regulation of inflammation and the maintenance and stability of cell membranes. They're called "essential" because the body is incapable of making them, so we must get these nutrients through our diets and/or supplementation. While several fatty acids are beneficial to human health, only two of them are essential: **linoleic acid** (LA) and **alpha-linolenic acid** (ALA). Some fatty acids are referred to as "conditionally essential," meaning that they can become essential under circumstances where a person's body lacks the ability to make them from the "parent" EFAs. Examples include **docosahexaenoic acid** (DHA), **eicosapentaenoic acid** (EPA), **arachidonic acid** (AA), and **gamma-linolenic acid** (GLA).

There are two categories of EFAs: **omega-3** (n-3 or ω-3) and **omega-6** (n-6 or ω-6). Omega-3 and omega-6 fatty acids are classified as **polyunsaturated fatty acids** (PUFAs) because they have more than one carbon-to-carbon double bond in their molecular structures. (Fatty acids with no double or triple bonds between any two carbon atoms are **saturated**, and fatty acids with only one carbon-to-carbon double bond in the entire molecule are **monounsaturated**.) Alpha-linolenic acid is an omega-3 fatty acid from which other, non-essential omega-3 fatty acids can be synthesized. Similarly, linoleic acid is an omega-6 fatty acid from which other omega-6 fatty acids can be made by the body.

Excess omega-6 fatty acids in the diet interfere with the metabolism of omega-3 fatty acids, mainly because they compete for the same enzymes. A high proportion of omega-6 to omega-3 fatty acids in the diet shifts the physiological state in the tissues toward the pathogenesis of many diseases.[28] Typical Western diets have a ratio of omega-6 to omega-3 fatty acids greater than 10:1, with some as high as 30:1, and the average ratio of omega-6 to omega-3 in such diets is 15:1 to 16.7:1.[29]

While it has been established that consuming too many omega-6 fatty acids in proportion to omega-3 fatty acids can lead to health problems,[29] the optimal ratio of omega-6 to omega-3 fatty acids is a matter of debate because it can vary among individuals, depending on their genetic makeup,[30] stage of life (e.g., infancy),[31] and whether or not they have any diseases or conditions that are affected by the fatty acid composition of the body.[29] In general, though, a ratio of 4:1 to 1:1 (ω-6:ω-3) is often recommended for healthy adults.

A comprehensive discussion of omega-3 and -6 fatty acids is beyond the scope of this book, but if you'd like to learn more about their roles in human physiology and their potential for healing a variety of ailments, please refer to my website (robynphelan.com) for links to additional resources. The remainder of this chapter is about the importance of essential fatty acids to the health and appearance of the skin. You'll also find information about several noteworthy botanical oils that may prove to be the missing link to your skin care woes.

EFAs Are Nature's Moisturizers

As mentioned in an earlier chapter, the keratinocytes in the stratum corneum layer of the epidermis are situated within an extracellular lipid matrix, which is responsible for the skin's function as a protective barrier. Excessive transepidermal water loss, a common occurrence in aging skin, is one of the manifestations of an essential fatty acid deficiency[32] and is directly related to the EFA content of stratum corneum lipids.[33] Linoleic acid (omega-6) is the most abundant PUFA in the epidermis, and it's an important component of two lipids found in the stratum corneum: acylceramide and acylglucosylceramide. Ceramides are a type of lipid composed of a fatty acid and sphingosine, an 18-carbon amino alcohol with an unsaturated hydrocarbon chain. The presence of linoleic acid in the ceramides of the stratum corneum is crucial for maintaining the permeability barrier function of the epidermis.[33] Skin-related symptoms of an essential fatty acid deficiency have been shown to respond favorably to both oral and topical use of oils rich in linoleic acid.[34-35]

EFAs and Collagen Synthesis

Eicosapentaenoic acid is an omega-3 fatty acid that is found in fish oil and is frequently accompanied in nature by docosahexaenoic acid. Fish oil is obviously not a botanical product, but it's worth mentioning because the fish themselves don't produce EPA and DHA; they get it from the algae that they consume (unless they're farm-raised and don't eat their natural diet). Consequently, plant-based omega-3 fatty acid supplements are popular among vegans and vegetarians. While neither EPA nor DHA are essential fatty acids, they may become essential in cases where there's a deficiency of ALA or where the body cannot make them efficiently from its supply of ALA. For example, it's suspected that women are better than men at converting ALA to EPA and DHA.[36]

In terms of skin health, topical application of EPA in particular shows promise as a means of both preventing the breakdown of collagen[37] and indirectly stimulating collagen synthesis by contributing to the synthesis of proteins that are necessary for building and repairing collagen.[38] One problem with EPA, however, is that both topical[39] and dietary[40] use have been observed to increase lipid peroxidation and decrease vitamin C and glutathione in mouse epidermis, and the same is likely to be true in human epidermis.[41]

In addition, a study involving 25 women of varying ages indicates that long-term use of fish oil supplements increases lipid peroxidation and may lead to a vitamin E deficiency.[42] The reason for the potential deficiency is that EPA is a so-called "long-chain" omega-3 PUFA and is chemically unstable due to the high number of double bonds. Vitamin E is a lipid-soluble antioxidant that mediates free radical damage caused by the oxidation of PUFAs. Unfortunately, high intakes of purified fish oil (in which the natural antioxidants have been removed) can raise the body's demand for vitamin E. The researchers warn that although fish oil capsules contain synthetic vitamin E to enhance the shelf life of the product, the amount of vitamin E in each capsule may be inadequate to guard against tissue damage caused by ROS.

In a 2011 paper about omega-3 fatty acids as photoprotective macronutrients, the authors state that "cosupplementation of n-3 PUFA with antioxidants may be necessary to counteract potential increases in oxidative stress as a result of n-3 PUFA peroxidation; whereas this seems reasonable, it is not certain, and little is actually known regarding the appropriate ingested n-3 PUFA/antioxidant balance in humans."[43] Despite the uncertainty regarding the proper balance, it's well-established that dietary antioxidants are important for protecting the skin from UV radiation,[44-48] but they shouldn't be relied upon in lieu of topical sunscreens. Incidentally, topical sunscreen has been shown[49] to repair collagen and elastin damage (albeit in mice).

EFAs and Skin Lightening

Aside from stimulating collagen synthesis and protecting the skin from UV damage, the fading of dark spots caused by increased melanin production is another benefit for which topical vitamin C is known, and it's one that can be addressed with topical linoleic and alpha-linolenic acids instead.[50] Based on the referenced study, the implication is that when applied to the skin, oils containing high levels of these fatty acids can inhibit melanin production and increase the rate of cell turnover in the stratum corneum, thereby giving the skin a more youthful appearance.

Why Botanical Oils?

Botanical oils are among the most powerful and cost-effective natural anti-aging treatments, even though some of them are on the pricey side. With oils, however, it's important to remember that a little bit goes a long way. A few drops is all you need to cover your face and neck, and when you see what they can do for your skin, don't be surprised if you end up ditching your tiny jar of thirty-dollar night cream in favor of a tiny bottle of oil that is available at a fraction of the price and will last much longer.

Another thing that makes oils wallet-friendly is that most of them can be used alone to get fantastic results. In other words, there's no need to combine an oil with other anti-aging ingredients to make something special because each of the oils described in this book is special enough by itself (although sea buckthorn oil in particular should be diluted with another oil because its dark color can temporarily stain the skin). If you're feeling overwhelmed with all of the possibilities and challenges when it comes to making your own anti-aging skin care products, then keep things simple. Once you see how well botanical oils perform on their own, you may not feel the need to put anything else on your face, including makeup. (But don't skip the sunscreen!)

When you begin researching botanical oils of interest, you'll inevitably come across people who have shared their personal experiences on forums and blogs, as well as in reviews on sites wherever botanical oils are for sale. (Granted, some reviews on commercial sites might have been written by shills, but I trust that you're astute enough to know when someone's trying to manipulate you.) Many women who use oils have found that they were eventually able to quit using makeup because their skin started looking healthy and clear without it (i.e., they have experienced reductions in fine lines and wrinkles, as well as increased elasticity, decreased sagging, and the lightening or disappearance of age spots and acne scars).

Even though anecdotal evidence is far from scientific, I don't believe that it should be disregarded by default. Conducting formal research can cost anywhere from thousands to millions of dollars, and there's not much of a financial incentive for companies to study natural products because they're difficult to patent,[51-53] and they present several challenges from a logistics point of view.[54]

Just because no one has published any data regarding the merits of a particular botanical oil as an anti-aging solution doesn't mean that the product is ineffective. More than likely, data have been published regarding the merits of certain chemical compounds that are present in plant-based oils in general, so if you can find out exactly what's in them, you can search (see Chapter 12) for scientific papers about the use of specific compounds to treat wrinkles, stimulate collagen synthesis, lighten age spots, etc. You can then infer that any oils containing said compounds *may* be effective skin treatments. Following that, the best way to know if something will work for you personally is to try it and see what happens. (I realize that some medical conditions are too serious for self-treatment, but experimenting with skin care products is a fairly benign practice for otherwise healthy people.)

The Elephant in the Room

The major concern that most people have when presented with the idea of putting oil on their faces is, "Won't it cause my skin to break out?" The answer depends on the oil and the individual. Some oils are better for dry skin, while others are better for oily skin and acne-prone skin. As a matter of fact, many people who suffer from acne and/or oily skin are fond of the "oil cleanse method," which involves washing your face with oil, not soap or some other type of cleanser. There's a saying in chemistry that "like dissolves like,"[55] and it helps chemists remember what substances will dissolve easily in others. The failure of oil and water to mix is one example of this principle in action, and it's the reason that washing your face with oil may be better than using water. An oil-based cleanser can dissolve and remove oil build-up (and makeup) without irritating or drying your skin, unlike many water-based cleansers that contain detergents (e.g., sodium lauryl sulfate and related chemicals) that can wash away your skin's acid mantle. Interestingly, the third and fourth ingredients listed on the label of the classic (some might even say "old school") facial cleanser, Noxzema®, are linseed oil (flaxseed oil) and soybean oil. Noxzema also contains water and an emulsifier to make the oils mix with the water, but the point is that oil is being used as a major ingredient in a cleanser.

The second concern that people have with oil is, "I don't want my face to look like an oil slick." Again, whether or not this will happen depends on the oil and the individual. Some oils are not greasy like you might expect them to be. They get absorbed into the skin quickly and leave it feeling softer and more elastic. After waiting a few minutes, you can apply makeup without it sliding off your face. Depending on the oil that you choose, you can achieve either a "matte" or a "dewey" look. If you find that your skin looks a bit too shiny after applying the oil, pat it with a tissue or give it a dusting of loose powder. You could also try different oils until you find one that gives you the look that you're going for right out of the bottle.

Alternatively, you could use your favorite oil only before going to sleep. After washing your face with the cleanser of your choice, pat your skin dry with a clean towel, and then pour a pea-sized amount (or less) of oil into your palm. Spread it between your hands, and dab it over your face. Gently massage the oil into your skin, including your neck and upper chest area (you may need a few more drops of oil). When you wake up the next day, your skin should be feeling soft and smooth, and you may find that you don't need to wash your face again at this time. You can just apply your sunscreen and makeup as usual.

Botanical Oils for Ageless Skin

While there are over 80 botanical oils that can be used in skin care products, I've chosen to include information about only those oils which I believe offer the greatest anti-aging properties. Again, some of them are more expensive than others, but they usually have one or more outstanding qualities that make them worth every penny. I should also clarify that by "botanical oils," I'm referring to fruit and vegetable oils that are obtained from the plant's pulp or seeds. These oils are commonly used as "carrier oils" ("fixed oils") for another group of botanical oils called "essential oils," although they can be used in isolation with remarkable benefits.

Another clarification that should be made relates to fatty acids. In biological systems, fatty acids normally occur in the form of triglycerides. A **triglyceride** is a type of ester[56] consisting of one molecule of glycerol (also known as glycerin) attached to three fatty acid molecules. Glycerin is one of the compounds produced during **saponification**, the chemical reaction that produces soap from fats and lye. Industrially, glycerin is often removed from the soap and sold separately. This is unfortunate for consumers because glycerin softens the skin and helps it retain moisture.[57] Some handmade soaps haven't been stripped of their glycerin, so they tend to be more skin-friendly than their mass-produced counterparts. The quality of such soaps, however, varies according to the fats and oils that were chosen, but that's a topic for another book. When discussing botanical oils in the following pages, I refer to specific fatty acids that are present in the oils, but you should be aware that they exist predominantly in triglyceride form, not the so-called "free fatty acid" form. This is an important distinction because in your research, you may come across studies where free fatty acids were used topically and were shown to behave differently on the skin than products containing the triglyceride forms.

If you're not aware of this nuance, it may cause you to avoid a potentially beneficial natural product for the wrong reasons. For example, pure oleic acid is known to be **comedogenic** (i.e., it clogs pores), but many botanical oils containing oleic acid (in triglyceride form) are non-comedogenic. If you have oily or acne-prone skin, though, it's best to use oils that are low in oleic acid, but you need not avoid it completely, nor can you. It's a natural component of human sebum.

Whether triglycerides are applied topically or ingested, the skin and body can metabolize them to produce the free fatty acids as necessary.[58] As such, it's more convenient to refer to a specific fatty acid by name, rather than a triglyceride, which may contain up to three different fatty acids. The fatty acid profiles of botanical oils that you'll see in books and other publications state the percentages (usually as a range) of fatty acids found in the oils, but these numbers don't correspond to free fatty acids. The relative amounts of each fatty acid found in the triglycerides of a botanical oil are determined by chemically breaking apart the triglycerides to obtain the free fatty acids. After isolating the fatty acids (usually in their esterified forms), chemists can analyze them to find out which ones are present and in what quantities.

Anti-Aging Botanical Oils

ANDIROBA

Andiroba oil comes from the nuts of the andiroba tree (also known as crabwood tree), which is found in parts of Africa and South America. The unrefined oil is brown and murky, while the refined oil has a golden yellow color and a mild, fruity aroma. Andiroba oil is emollient and penetrates the skin easily. It contains compounds with anti-inflammatory activity and can be used topically to treat acne, dry or cracked skin, eczema, psoriasis, muscular aches, and swelling. In addition, andiroba oil is a natural insect repellant and is particularly effective at warding off mosquitoes. If you've been dissatisfied with the performance (or smell) of citronella candles, then try a candle made with andiroba oil instead. (They may be hard to find in the United States, but if you can get some of the oil itself, maybe you could make your own andiroba candles.)

The fatty acid profile of refined andiroba oil is: oleic acid (50.5%), palmitic acid (28%), linoleic acid (9%), stearic acid (8.1%), arachidic acid (1.2%), palmitoleic acid (1%).[59]

ARGAN

Argan oil is pressed from the kernels found inside the nuts of the argan tree, which grows exclusively in Morocco. Both the traditional and semi-industrialized extraction processes[60] are more labor-intensive than those for other oils, hence the high cost of argan oil. The effort is worth the trouble, however, since the chemical composition of argan oil makes for a nutritious food[60-61] and a highly prized skin and hair care product. Refined argan oil is used for cosmetics and personal care products, whereas the food-grade oil is used for culinary purposes. Production of the latter involves roasting the argan kernels, giving the resulting oil a nutty aroma that may be undesirable for skin care applications, so the cosmetic-grade oil is extracted without first roasting the kernels. Alternatively, the virgin argan oil may be deodorized later for cosmetic use. Deodorized virgin argan oil is a medium-viscosity oil with a golden color. It's very moisturizing and penetrates the skin quickly. The high vitamin E content (mostly in the form of gamma-tocopherol) not only gives the oil a long shelf life, but it also provides long-term antioxidant capacity for the skin, since tocopherols are incorporated into cell membranes.[61]

The fatty acid profile of argan oil is: oleic acid (43-50%), linoleic acid (29.3-37%), palmitic acid (10-15%), stearic acid (4.3-7.2%).[62]

AVOCADO

Avocado oil is cold-pressed from the pulp, rather than the pit, of the avocado fruit. Its emerald green color is due to the presence of chlorophyll. The unrefined version, used mainly in food preparation, smells like avocado and contains a higher nutrient content than cosmetic-grade avocado oil, which is a pale yellow, odorless product that is extracted at elevated temperatures. Be skeptical of any claims that avocado oil is rich in vitamin C or any of the B vitamins. While it's true that the pulp contains vitamins B and C and that the oil is obtained from the pulp, the water is removed from the pulp by evaporation before cold pressing the oil. Therefore, any water-soluble nutrients are left behind as solids mixed with the pulp and do not make their way into the oil, where they would not dissolve. By contrast, fat-soluble compounds such as vitamin E (in the form of mixed tocopherols), vitamin A (in the forms of alpha- and beta-carotene), phytosterols, and sterolins are all present in avocado oil.

Avocado oil is emollient and penetrates the skin well, although not as quickly as other oils because of its medium to thick viscosity and high oleic acid content relative to linoleic acid. The fatty acid profile of unrefined avocado oil is: oleic acid (68.6%), linoleic acid (15.4%), palmitic acid (11.3%), palmitoleic acid (3.5%), stearic acid (1.1%).[63]

Avocado oil is a great oil to use in soap making because it contains many **unsaponifiables**, or compounds that don't participate in the saponification reaction. Consequently, soaps made with avocado oil leave the skin feeling soft and moisturized, as if avocado oil itself were applied directly to the skin.

Avocado oil is also great as a pre-shampoo treatment for dry or damaged hair. (Applying this oil to clean, damp hair before blow-drying tends to weigh it down too much, making the hair look flat.) By the way, if you find that a certain oil isn't quite right for your face, you could always try it in your hair before giving up on it and feeling like you wasted your money. You could also try it on areas of skin that are prone to dryness, such as elbows and heels, but if you have severely dry elbows or heels, you might be better off using a botanical "butter" like mango butter, shea butter, or cupuaçu butter.

BAOBAB

Baobab trees are native to Africa and parts of India. All parts of the tree are used locally for a variety of applications, but the oil from the seeds of the baobab fruit is becoming increasingly popular as a cosmetic and nutraceutical ingredient for the global market. Cold pressed baobab oil is a highly emollient, golden yellow oil with a nutty aroma and a medium viscosity. It soaks into the skin quickly and won't clog pores. Baobab oil is a good choice for aging skin because it can increase the skin's elasticity[64] and, like many oils, reduce the appearance of fine lines and wrinkles. Baobab oil also contains significant amounts of sterols and tocopherols.[65-66]

The fatty acid profile of baobab oil is: oleic acid (30-40%), linoleic acid (24-34%), palmitic acid (18-30), stearic acid (2-8%), linolenic acid (0.5-3%).[66]

BLACK RASPBERRY

Black raspberry seed oil is a lightweight oil whose color ranges from pale gold to pale green. Like other berry seed oils, it contains significant amounts of the two essential fatty acids: linoleic acid (53.5%) and alpha-linolenic acid (31.2%).[67] The high vitamin E content of black raspberry seed oil contributes to its stable shelf life (one year) and its ability to provide antioxidant activity in the skin. It's tocopherol content isn't as high as that of red raspberry seed oil, however.[67]

BLACKBERRY

Blackberry seed oil is rich in antioxidants, although it doesn't have as much vitamin E as red or black raspberry seed oil.[67] The Marion blackberry variety has more linoleic and oleic acids, but less alpha-linolenic acid, than the raspberry seed oils.[67] Blackberry seed oil's fatty acid profile is: linoleic acid (54-60%), oleic acid (15-19%), alpha-linolenic acid (15-20%).[68]

Blackberry seed oil has a greenish color and a mild scent. Because it's one of the most expensive oils, it is often used at lower concentrations, although it can be applied directly to the skin. If you happen to come across "cheap" blackberry seed oil, it's possible that it might have been diluted with some other oil, even if it doesn't say so on the label. I haven't found any published examples concerning blackberry seed oil in particular, but adulteration is an unfortunate reality in the oil industry,[69-71] and it's something to be aware of when sourcing oils for your skin care products and dietary needs. Also be mindful of oils or other perishable ingredients that are "on sale." This could mean that the ingredient is nearing the end of its shelf life.

BLUEBERRY

Blueberry seed oil is a greenish-yellow oil with a mild fruity scent and a light viscosity. It absorbs quickly without leaving a greasy afterfeel and is a good choice for people with oily or sensitive skin. Although blueberry seed oil contains a variety of antioxidants, one study suggests that its oxidative stability is due to the oil's tocopherol content and not any of the phenolic antioxidants that were quantified.[72] This oil, however, doesn't contain nearly the amount of vitamin E that red raspberry seed oil does,[73] and its shelf life is only half as long.[74] The fatty acid profile of blueberry seed oil is: linoleic acid (38-43%), alpha-linolenic acid (28-33%), oleic acid (18-23%), palmitic acid (3-5%).[75]

BORAGE

Borage oil (or borage seed oil) is known for being exceptionally high in gamma-linolenic acid (GLA), a conditionally essential fatty acid that human skin cannot synthesize from its precursor, linoleic acid (LA). In young and healthy bodies, a liver enzyme called **delta-6-desaturase** (commonly written as Δ^6desaturase) converts dietary LA to GLA, which then makes its way to the skin through the bloodstream. In elderly or otherwise unhealthy people (e.g., diabetics), delta-6-desaturase activity may be impaired.[76] Taking borage oil internally bypasses the metabolic step that forms GLA from LA and may compensate for health conditions where essential fatty acid metabolism is known to be suboptimal.[77-78]

When used externally, borage oil is purported to moisturize and soften the skin, increase its elasticity, and encourage cell turnover. The fatty acid profile of borage oil is: linoleic acid (35-42%), gamma-linolenic acid (20%), oleic acid (15-20%), palmitic acid (9%), stearic acid (3-5%), eicosenoic acid (3-5%).[79] Unfortunately, it's an expensive oil with a six-month shelf life. To make it last longer, you can refrigerate it and add vitamin E or a stabilizing oil, such as red raspberry or meadowfoam. It's also important to be aware that borage oil may contain pyrrolizidine alkaloids, which are toxic to the liver.[80] Therefore, if you're going to use this oil, make sure that it has been certified free of pyrrolizidine alkaloids.

CAMELLIA

Camellia oil is cold pressed from the seeds of *Camellia japonica*, a flowering tree native to Asia. This oil is also called "Japanese camellia oil" or "Tsubaki oil" and should not be confused with the oils derived from other camellia varieties, such as "tea oil camellia" (from *Camellia sinensis*) and "tea seed oil" (from *Camellia oleifera*).[81] The latter two oils should also not be confused with "tea tree oil," an inedible essential oil from the tea tree, which grows in Australia and is often used as a topical treatment for a variety of dermatological conditions, including acne.[82] Unlike other botanical oils, pure tea tree oil is available at chain drug stores throughout the U.S. Oddly enough, you won't find it anywhere near the acne treatment products. Look for it in the vitamin aisle. Tea tree oil smells strongly of camphor, so it's best to use it at night after washing your face and applying your botanical oil of choice. Simply dab it onto the affected areas with a cotton swab. As with all oils, a little bit goes a long way, so you shouldn't need to use more than one swab for several spots.

Getting back to Japanese camellia oil, it's very high in oleic acid (>80%) and low in linoleic acid (1-5%). It's also relatively low in tocopherols and sterols.[83] However, this pale yellow oil is an effective emollient, and it penetrates the skin easily. In terms of anti-aging skin care, it has been shown to improve skin hydration and to inhibit one of the matrix metalloproteinases (MMP-1), as well as to promote the synthesis of human type I procollagen.[83] (There are several types of collagen in the human body. Types I and III are found in the skin. Procollagen is a precursor to collagen.) Tsubaki oil is one of the beauty secrets of the Japanese Geishas, while the other camellia oils are mainly used for culinary purposes (although they can be used for skin and hair care, too).

CARROT

Carrot seed oil is cold pressed from the seeds of *Daucus carota* (wild carrot or Queen Anne's lace) and should not be confused with "Helio Carrot" or "carrot seed essential oil." Some vendors will reference "carrot oil," leaving it up to the consumer to figure out which type of carrot oil it is. All of them have beneficial properties for the skin, but they have different applications and should be used accordingly. Unrefined carrot seed oil has a golden or brassy color, a strong herbal odor, and a medium viscosity. This non-greasy oil absorbs quickly and has the following fatty acid profile: oleic acid (68.4%), linoleic acid (10.8%), alpha-linolenic acid (0.2%). It also contains beta-carotene and several sterols.[84]

CRANBERRY

Unrefined cranberry seed oil is cold pressed from the seeds of cranberries. This oil has a unique balance of omega-3, -6, and -9 fatty acids and the highest tocotrienol content of any botanical oil known thus far.[85] Cranberry seed oil is golden yellow and has a mild scent. This medium-viscosity oil quickly penetrates the skin without leaving a greasy afterfeel. Due to its high vitamin E content, it has a stable shelf life and can be used to extend the shelf lives of other oils. The fatty acid profile of cranberry seed oil is: linoleic acid (37.68%), alpha-linolenic acid (30.09%), oleic acid (25.30%), palmitic acid (5.38%).[86]

CUCUMBER

Cucumber seed oil comes from the cleaned and dried seeds of cucumbers. This yellow oil is highly moisturizing and absorbs easily. It does smell a bit like cucumber, but the odor goes away once the oil has penetrated the skin. The same is usually true of other oils that have a mild aroma. Cucumber seed oil is among the oils with the highest amounts of linoleic acid and is a good choice for dry skin, as well as maturing skin and acne-prone skin. The fatty acid profile of cucumber seed oil is: linoleic acid (60-68%), oleic acid (14-20%), palmitic acid (9-13%), stearic acid (6-9%).[87]

EVENING PRIMROSE

Like borage oil, evening primrose oil is notably high in gamma-linolenic acid. It is often used as a nutritional supplement to reduce or eliminate the symptoms of premenstrual syndrome (PMS). Evening primrose oil is also very high in linoleic acid while being very low in oleic acid, which makes it a good choice for all skin types. This golden yellow oil absorbs quickly and leaves the skin feeling soft and supple. The fatty acid profile of evening primrose oil is: linoleic acid (68-76%), gamma-linolenic acid (10%), oleic acid (6-10%), palmitic acid (5-7%), stearic acid (1-3%).[88]

GRAPESEED

The seeds of grapes are considered waste products in the wine and grape juice industry, but they're useful in the cosmetics industry for making lotions and creams that feature the cold-pressed oil as a base. Grapeseed oil is a low-viscosity, light green oil with either a faint odor or a strong one, depending on the source. Different grape varieties, such as chardonnay and Riesling, produce seed oils with slightly different properties. Grapeseed oil absorbs quickly and leaves a silky, non-greasy afterfeel. It's one of the least expensive oils and can usually be found in grocery stores, since it's also used for cooking. The fatty acid profile of grapeseed oil is: linoleic acid (71.7-73.1%), oleic acid (15.4-15.6%), palmitic acid (7.2-8.5%), stearic acid (3.8-3.9%).[89]

HAZELNUT

Hazelnut oil is cold pressed from the nuts of hazel trees or shrubs. Different hazel varieties offer different fatty acid profiles. Chilean hazelnut oil,[90] for example, contains much more palmitoleic acid and less oleic acid than American hazelnut oil.[91] Palmitoleic acid is an omega-7 fatty acid that is naturally present in human sebum and acts as an antimicrobial.[92] Chilean hazelnut oil is light in color and nearly odorless. It's highly emollient and penetrates the skin quickly.

HEMP

Hemp oil is cold pressed from the seeds of industrially grown *Cannabis sativa*. Although industrial hemp is related to marijuana, it contains only trace amounts (less than 10 parts per million, or ppm) of the psychoactive compound, tetrahydrocannabinol (THC). Consuming hemp oil and other hemp foods poses no risk of intoxication or other detrimental side effects associated with THC. In addition, hemp oil and hemp foods are extremely unlikely to cause anyone to fail a urine test for marijuana. When used topically, any THC in hemp oil is not absorbed through the skin.[93]

The fatty acid profile of hemp oil makes it a valuable food and skin care ingredient, as it contains omega-6 and omega-3 fatty acids in the "ideal" ratio of 3:1.[94] One tablespoon of Nutiva Organic Cold-Pressed Hemp Oil contains 7.0 g linoleic acid (LA), 2.5 g alpha-linolenic acid (ALA), 500 mg gamma-linolenic acid (GLA), and 250 mg of stearidonic acid (SDA), along with 2.0 g of oleic acid.[95] In terms of percentage ranges, hemp oil contains 54-57% LA, 16-20% ALA, 2-4% GLA, 0.5-1.5% SDA, 10-13% oleic acid, and 0.5% eicosaenoic acid.[96]

Hemp oil has a bit less than half the amount of GLA as evening primrose oil (EPO), a popular natural remedy for PMS. Premenstrual syndrome is commonly thought to be caused by a hormonal imbalance, but many women who experience PMS have normal hormone levels. An alternate explanation for the physical and psychological disturbances associated with PMS is that "PMS is a mild abnormality of essential fatty acid (EFA) metabolism" in which the conversion of LA to GLA may be impaired.[97] Daily supplementation with GLA may help alleviate symptoms of PMS. The essential fatty acids found in hemp oil, EPO, and other oils can also help reduce appetite and food cravings while increasing energy and metabolism.[153] Since EPO supplements are expensive and do not provide the appropriate balance of omega-3 and omega-6 fatty acids, hemp oil is a cost-effective and versatile alternative that can address nutritional, therapeutic, and cosmetic needs.

Unrefined hemp oil is light green and has a medium viscosity. It looks similar to olive oil but has quite a different odor and flavor, which are both often described as "nutty" or "grassy" (no pun intended). The taste is not to everyone's liking, but it can be masked if combined with olive oil or another flavorful oil like roasted walnut oil. The refined version is normally used for cosmetic purposes, but the unrefined oil can be used as well, as long as you don't mind the greenish tint that it will give to lotions, creams, soaps, and other products. Although hemp oil is available in softgel form, purchasing the pure oil in bulk and finding a way to swallow it without grimacing is much cheaper. (Actually, it's not that bad. I drink a tablespoon of the stuff every day, and I have no regrets.)

MACADAMIA NUT

Like Chilean hazelnut oil, macadamia nut oil has an appreciable quantity of palmitoleic acid. If you research the skin benefits of macadamia nut oil, you'll find no shortage of beauty blogs and commercial websites that mention, without supporting evidence, something to the effect of, "Palmitoleic acid in the skin declines with age," implying that topical use of macadamia nut oil can restore the amount of palmitoleic acid in the skin to youthful levels. Statements regarding the decreased level of palmitoleic acid in mature skin are inconsistent with the findings of Eun Ju Kim and colleagues, who determined that "palmitoleic acid and oleic acid were increased in aged skin by 67% and 22%, respectively, compared with those in young skin."[98] In addition, they observed that linoleic, palmitic, and stearic acids were less prevalent in aged skin than in young skin. The unsubstantiated hype about palmitoleic acid in macadamia nut oil is also inconsistent with research[99] that has identified the oxidative degradation of palmitoleic acid in middle-aged and elderly skin as the culprit in what many people refer to as "old person smell."

Although macadamia nut oil is often recommended (by people who sell macadamia nut oil, of course) for mature skin, it's not clear to me why that would be the case, since it consists primarily of oleic acid (50-67%), followed by palmitoleic acid (14-22%).[100] Having said that, macadamia nut oil does make the skin feel soft and smooth. It can also be used to moisturize dry, damaged hair without weighing it down (if applied to damp hair before blow-drying). It has a light amber color, a medium viscosity, and a nutty aroma. Seed oils (especially the refined ones) don't typically smell like the plants from which they came, but there are a few exceptions, and macadamia nut oil is one of them. If you apply this oil to your skin, you might smell more like a macadamia nut than an old person, but only time will tell.

MARACUJÁ

Maracujá oil comes from the seeds of passion fruit, a plant that is native to tropical and subtropical climates. "Maracujá" is the Portuguese word for passion fruit, and some passion fruit oil is labeled as such because the oil is often sourced from Brazil, where Portuguese is the official language. When looking for Maracujá oil, you may find two different varieties for sale: *Passiflora edulis* and *Passiflora incarnata*. The former species is native to South America, while the latter is native to the southern United States. Maracujá oil's fatty acid content features approximately 73% linoleic acid and 14% oleic acid.[101] The seeds of *Passiflora edulis* contain a compound called **piceatannol**, which has been shown to inhibit melanin synthesis[102] and may thus be a safer way to treat hyperpigmentation than potentially carcinogenic drugs like hydroquinone, arbutin, and kojic acid.[103]

At the time of this writing, a small (1.7 fl oz) bottle of Maracujá Oil from Tarte Cosmetics will set you back

$46.00.[104] This is a shining example of retail markup, to which I encourage you not to fall prey. If you'd like to try maracujá oil, then you can purchase roughly the same quantity (2 fl oz) from a wholesale supplier like Natural Sourcing, LLC (fromnaturewithlove.com) for a modest seven dollars and fifty cents.[105]

MEADOWFOAM

Meadowfoam seed oil comes from *Limnanthes alba*, a flowering plant that is native to California and Oregon. The unusual fatty acid profile of meadowfoam seed oil places this natural product in a league of its own. The dominant fatty acids of most plant seed oils are oleic and linoleic acids, but meadowfoam seed oil has neither. Instead, it has about 60% *cis*-5-eicosenoic acid, 19% *cis*-5-*cis*-13-docosadienoic acid, 10% *cis*-13-docosenoic acid (also known as erucic acid), and 8% *cis*-5-docosenoic acid.[106-107]

One of the most celebrated properties of meadowfoam seed oil is that it's more stable than any other vegetable oil.[108] The oxidative stability of meadowfoam seed oil is not due to its vitamin E content as one might expect, but rather the inherent stabilities of its fatty acids,[106,109] whose molecular structures contain one or two carbon-to-carbon double bonds in locations that make them less susceptible to oxidation than if they were in other positions.

Meadowfoam seed oil has a light golden color and a faint, pleasant odor. It's slightly viscous and does not get absorbed completely. For this reason, meadowfoam seed oil forms a moisturizing barrier that protects against transepidermal water loss. Its tendency to stay on the skin, in addition to its lubricating property, is why this oil is sometimes used as a substitute for dimethicone (a type of silicone) in products that aim to be 100% natural. Another noteworthy property of meadowfoam oil is that its performance in skin and hair care products is similar to that of jojoba oil.[108] Since jojoba oil (which is actually a wax ester, not an oil) tends to be expensive, meadowfoam seed oil is an economical alternative.

MORINGA

Moringa oil is obtained from the seeds of *Moringa oleifera*, a tree that grows in Africa and parts of Asia. It is sometimes referred to as a "drumstick tree." The leaves are edible and contain several vitamins and trace minerals.[110] Because moringa leaves are an excellent source of vitamin C, the seed oil is often touted as being rich in vitamin C as well, but this is a marketing falsehood that gets perpetuated from one resource to another in the absence of fact checking and critical thinking.

After contacting two companies that sell moringa oil and asking how it's possible that this oil contains a water-soluble vitamin, they both replied to me with something to the effect of, "That was a mistake on our website. We'll let our writers know about the issue and have them correct it." (Sure, blame the underlings.) The moral of the story is that although some companies offer high-quality ingredients for your DIY projects, they may not be very knowledgeable about what they're selling, so you can't always rely on their product descriptions.

Moringa oil is a pale yellow oil with a light viscosity and a mild, nutty aroma. The oil can be used for culinary or beauty purposes and is also known as "ben oil" and "behen oil" because of its behenic acid content. If you decide to consume moringa oil, be advised that dietary behenic acid can raise cholesterol, despite the fact that it is poorly absorbed by the body.[111]

The fatty acid profile of moringa oil is: oleic acid (71.6%), palmitic acid (6.34%), behenic acid (6.21%), stearic acid (5.70%), arachidic acid (3.52%), eicosenoic acid (2.24%), linoleic acid (0.77%).[112] Interestingly, the saturated fatty acid content of moringa oil makes for a potential source of biodiesel.[113]

POMEGRANATE

Thinning of the epidermis and a reduced cell turnover rate are characteristic of aging skin. Pomegranate seed oil's claim to fame is that it can not only increase cell turnover by stimulating the proliferation of keratinocytes, but it can also thicken the epidermis without resulting in "disordered differentiation" (i.e., increased cell size).[114] In addition, the fatty acid profile of pomegranate seed oil is unusual in that the primary fatty acid is **punicic acid**, and the quantities of oleic and linoleic acids are relatively low. Punicic acid is an omega-5 fatty acid that has been shown to inhibit the proliferation of breast cancer.[115]

And now for the bad news: pomegranate seed oil is a heavy, sticky oil that doesn't penetrate the skin very well. It also has a strong odor that can't be masked by essential oils. Therefore, you'd probably want to use it only sparingly in your skin care formulations.

RED RASPBERRY

It's hard to imagine that any oil could be pressed from a raspberry seed, but somebody found a way to do it. The only problem is that it takes 80 pounds of seeds to produce a gallon of oil,[116] which is one reason for its relatively high cost. The benefits are worth it, though. This golden yellow oil has a light viscosity and absorbs quickly, leaving the skin very soft. It's an excellent choice for normal, oily, or combination skin but may not be suitable for very dry skin. It's also what I would call a "matte" oil in that it doesn't leave a sheen on your skin like other oils do. When used on damp hair before blowing it dry, a few drops of this oil can provide softness and bounce. Red raspberry seed oil smells faintly of raspberries, but it's not a fragrance oil per se. The scent dissipates when the oil has been completely absorbed into the skin.

Red raspberry seed oil is known for its potential to protect the skin against both UVA and UVB rays. Its broad spectrum protection is comparable to that of titanium dioxide, and it has a natural SPF ranging from 28-50.[117] While this property makes it a good oil to use as a cosmetic base for sun protection products, the pure oil should not be relied upon as a sunscreen, nor should it be labeled as an active ingredient in sunscreens. In order for any product to be sold as a sunscreen, the Food and Drug Administration (FDA) requires that it be tested through a certified laboratory. If you're tempted to make a sunscreen for your own personal use, be aware that the only way to know its SPF value is to have it formally tested, which costs a lot more than you probably want to spend.

The total tocopherol content of red raspberry seed oil is approximately eight times higher than that of blueberry seed oil.[73] Due to its rich vitamin E content, red raspberry seed oil can be used to extend the shelf lives of more fragile oils. Even though red raspberry seed oil is a "preservative" in the sense that it can improve the oxidative stability of other cosmetic ingredients, it should not be used as a "natural preservative" to guard against contamination by bacteria. The same is true for other oils that are high in vitamin E.

The fatty acid profile of red raspberry seed oil is: linoleic acid (50-60%), oleic acid (12-16%), alpha-linolenic acid (19-27%), palmitic acid (2-4%).[118]

RICE BRAN

Rice bran oil is extracted from the bran and germ of brown rice. This pale yellow oil leaves a silky afterfeel and is very moisturizing. It's most notable quality is that it contains gamma-oryzanol (γ-oryzanol), which is a mixture of ferulic acid esters of sterol and triterpene alcohols.[119-120] Gamma-oryzanol occurs in rice bran oil at a concentration of 1-2%[121] and is a natural antioxidant.[122] Rice bran oil has been shown to lower cholesterol in humans[123-124] and to ease the symptoms of menopause.[125] These physiological benefits have been attributed to γ-oryzanol.

The fatty acid profile of rice bran oil is: oleic acid (44.85%), linoleic acid (31.32%), palmitic acid (21.79%), stearic acid (1.86%).[126] The oil also contains less than 1% of alpha-linolenic acid. If you use rice bran oil as a food, it's important to make sure that you're getting enough omega-3 fatty acids in your diet to compensate for the high omega-6 fatty acid content of this otherwise healthy oil.

ROSE HIP

Rose hip seed oil (rosehip oil) is one of the most popular anti-aging botanical oils. Not only does it contain both essential fatty acids in significant quantities, it also contains **all-*trans*-retinoic acid** (tretinoin), which is a product of vitamin A (retinol) metabolism. Rose hip seed oil has been put on a pedestal because of its "vitamin A" content, but this is yet another marketing falsehood because vitamin A is found only in animal products. Any botanical oil that is said to contain "vitamin A" actually contains a precursor (e.g., beta-carotene) of vitamin A or, in the case of rosehip oil, a metabolite of vitamin A. The body must convert beta-carotene to the real vitamin A.

All-*trans*-retinoic acid is the active compound in rose hip seed oil that is responsible for its regenerative ability.[127] Tretinoin creams are used to treat a variety of skin conditions,[128] but they're available by prescription only, whereas rose hip seed oil is an over-the-counter (OTC) product. The prescription creams are known to cause undesirable side effects, but rose hip seed oil is gentle on the skin. To obtain rose hip seed oil with the highest cosmetic and therapeutic properties, it must be cold pressed. Extraction by way of organic solvents greatly reduces the amount of all-*trans*-retinoic acid in the oil yield.[127]

The unrefined oil has a dark orange color and a distinctive, but not unpleasant, odor. Using this oil in lotions or creams will give such products a yellow tint, unless you use the refined version, which is a pale yellow oil with a milder scent. Rose hip seed oil is more fragile than other oils and should be refrigerated in order to extend its shelf life. When using the oil in products that will not be refrigerated, it's best to incorporate **rosemary oleoresin extract** (rosemary oil extract or ROE) into the recipe to delay rancidity. In general, products containing botanical oils should also be kept in dark glass or opaque plastic containers to protect them from UV light.

The approximate fatty acid profile of cold pressed rose hip seed oil is: linoleic acid (48%), alpha-linolenic acid (26%), oleic acid (15%), palmitic acid (4.5%).[127]

SEA BUCKTHORN

Sea buckthorn (*Hippophae rhamnoides*) is a common shrub that grows in Europe and Asia. It produces orange berries that are traditionally used to make jams, jellies, syrups, juices, pies, fruit wines, and liquors. In the cosmetics industry, sea buckthorn oil is an active ingredient in lotions, creams, and anti-aging products. "Sea buckthorn oil" may refer to the oil obtained from either the seeds or pulp, or a combination of the two. It's important to know what you're buying because the fatty acid profile of sea buckthorn oil depends on whether it came from the seeds or the pulp.[129] If you're looking for essential fatty acids, you'll want to get the seed oil, which contains both linoleic and alpha-linolenic acids. If you're looking for monounsaturated and saturated fatty acids (palmitoleic acid and palmitic acid, respectively), they can be found in the pulp oil. Both the seed and pulp oils contain vitamin E (as tocopherols and tocotrienols), carotenoids, and phytosterols. Although sea buckthorn berries contain vitamin C,[130] neither the seed oil nor the pulp oil contain vitamin C. When sea buckthorn berries are cold pressed, the resulting liquid separates into three layers.[131] The top two layers are lipophilic ("fat loving"), while the bottom layer is hydrophilic ("water loving"). Because vitamin C is soluble in water and not oil, it remains in the hydrophilic layer.

Despite the long list of health benefits that sea buckthorn berries have to offer,[132] the oils present a few challenges when used topically. Sea buckthorn pulp/berry oil is a heavy, dark orange liquid that will temporarily stain the skin if used at full strength. The seed oil is light, non-greasy, and non-staining, but the combination of the two oils gives the best nutrient profile. Most oils that are sold as "sea buckthorn oil" contain either the pulp oil or the seed and pulp combination, and some of them could be mislabeled due to confusion or a genuine lack of in-depth product knowledge, as is common in the skin care industry. In addition, sea buckthorn oil from the pulp (or the pulp/seed combination) has an odor that many people find unpleasant. Last, but not least, this is an expensive oil. Just a quarter of an ounce will cost you about $10.00 or more. Another factor to consider is that sea buckthorn oil will solidify at cooler temperatures. If your main concern in choosing a botanical oil is the fatty acid profile, then there are other oils that provide both EFAs without the high cost, pungent odor, or risk of staining or solidifying.

STRAWBERRY

Strawberry seed oil contains about the same amount of linoleic and alpha-linolenic acids as cranberry seed oil, but only about half the amount of oleic acid.[87,133] This seed oil has a pale green color and a faint strawberry aroma (it's not strong enough to be used as a fragrance oil, though). It's highly emollient, non-greasy, and quick to absorb. If strawberry seed oil has any drawbacks, it's the price: a two-ounce bottle costs about $30.00 (fromnaturewithlove.com).

7

OIL EXTRACTION METHODS

When you're shopping for botanical oils, you'll often see information about how a particular oil was extracted, but this can be meaningless or confusing to the uninitiated. Retrieving the oil from seeds, nuts, kernels, and pulp can be done in several ways. The most common and most preferable method is cold pressing, during which the oil-containing materials are mechanically pressed while ensuring that the heat caused by friction doesn't rise above 120°F (about 49°C). It's important that the temperature remains at or below this level so that the oil's desirable properties are preserved. Too much heat may cause beneficial compounds in the oil to degrade.

Not all oils can be cold pressed, so they must be extracted by some other method. One such method is expeller pressing. This is similar to cold pressing, except that it's done at high pressure to maximize the yield of oil. Extraction under high pressure can result in temperatures exceeding 120°F, so the oil cannot be called "cold pressed" at that point. Some oils are extracted from their sources using solvents in order to make the procedure more efficient and less costly. The solvents are removed by evaporation under a vacuum, but there may be trace amounts of solvent left in the final product.

8
REFINED VS. UNREFINED OIL

In addition to being confused about extraction methods, another issue that may come up when shopping for botanical oils is whether or not you should use the refined or unrefined oil. Refined oils have been subjected to various processing methods in order to remove impurities, alter the color or texture, reduce or eliminate the odor, or stabilize the shelf life. Unrefined oils have been mechanically screen filtered to remove solid particles, and they haven't undergone any additional refinement. Consequently, they retain their original colors, odors, flavors, and nutrients.

Whether or not you should use refined or unrefined oils is a matter of personal preference and often has to do with the specific application. Refined oils are commonly preferred for commercial cosmetics and personal care

products, while unrefined oils are generally preferred*
for culinary use.

Many people who make their own skin care products
like to use unrefined oils because there are antioxidants
and other compounds in the oils that are good for the
skin but may be removed during the refining process.
Some plant oils and butters, however, have such strong
odors that using the refined versions is the way to go.
Unrefined shea butter, for example, has a pungent,
earthy odor that can't be covered up by fragrances. It also
has a grainy texture, whereas refined shea butter has a
smooth texture and no odor. (I recommend against
using shea butter on your face. It's greasy, shiny, and
pore-clogging. If you need to use a butter to create the
desired texture for your product, try refined cupuaçu
butter instead.)

*To be clear, some mass-produced cooking oils (soybean, corn, palm, etc.) are
highly refined and generally not preferred by the readership of this book.

9
VIRGIN VS. EXTRA VIRGIN OIL

The terms "virgin" and "extra virgin" apply specifically to olive oil. When it comes to other oils, there are no industry standards in the United States for labeling them as such. Coconut oil, for example, is often sold as "extra virgin," but there's no such thing; it's a marketing gimmick. There's no standard for "virgin" coconut oil, either, but the term is used to distinguish it from "coconut oil" (without the qualifier) that has been produced by a different method.[134] Virgin coconut oil is a white solid at room temperature, and it has a coconut flavor and aroma, whereas non-virgin coconut oil has no odor or taste. By the way, I don't recommend any form of coconut oil for the skin. A lot of people rave about it, but for some people, it can be very drying. It also has a tendency to clog pores. Virgin coconut oil is excellent for cooking and baking, though.

For most other botanical oils, the term "virgin" is used to indicate that the oil was produced from the first pressing of the nuts, seeds, or pulp and that it has not undergone any refinement. It may or may not have been mechanically screen filtered to remove solid particles. Virgin oils are considered to be unrefined.

10
WEIGHT VS. VOLUME AND WHY IT MATTERS

Some ingredients may be sold by weight, and others may be sold by volume. Most recipes call for ingredients (including liquids) to be measured by weight, so if you find that a particular liquid ingredient is for sale in fluid-ounce (fl oz) or milliliter (mL or ml) quantities, it's helpful to convert that number to a weight so that you know how much to order. Because different liquids have different densities, their weight per unit volume will not be the same. Therefore, you would need to do a quick calculation to see how many grams of the liquid in question correspond to the volume in which it's being sold.

To do the calculation, look up the "relative density" or "specific gravity" of the liquid. Let's use baobab oil as an example. Natural Sourcing, LLC (the parent company of From Nature With Love®) is one of the few companies that offer "spec sheets" for their products. Their specifications document for each botanical oil shows the relative density at 68°F (20°C), which is considered to be "room temperature." The spec sheet for baobab oil[135] states that the relative density is 0.85-0.99 g/ml.

Suppose that our recipe calls for 44 grams (g) of baobab oil, and we want to know its equivalent amount in fluid ounces. First, divide 44 g by 0.85 g/ml. (To be conservative, we'll use the lowest number of the range given.) The rounded answer is 52 ml. Now we need to convert that into fluid ounces. The easiest way to do that is to use an online calculator[136] to handle the conversion. In this case, the rounded result is 1.76 fl oz, so we would need to purchase a 2-oz container of baobab oil. Since 1.76 is so close to 2, it might be a good idea to buy more than 2 fl oz because some of the oil will get stuck to the insides of the container, and you might not end up with enough, unless you have a way to get every last drop. In general, it's also a good idea to have extra ingredients on hand in case you mess up and have to start over, or if you just want to experiment with them some more.

11

PRESERVATIVES AND ANTIOXIDANTS

Preservatives

If you're going to be making a product that contains water or other aqueous liquids, then using a preservative is absolutely necessary. In this context, "preservative" means any substance that prevents contamination by microorganisms (bacteria, fungi, yeasts, and molds). The most effective preservatives are synthetic, as opposed to natural. Although many natural products have antimicrobial activity, they're either too weak for the task at hand, or they would need to be used in quantities that are impractical. If you're opposed to using synthetic preservatives for whatever reason, then you have two options: stick with making products that don't require preservatives (e.g., make lotion bars instead of lotion), or use a "naturally derived" preservative (i.e., one whose ingredients are derived from natural products). An example of a naturally-derived preservative is Linatural MBS-1,[137-138] which is a mixture of propanediol, ethylhexyl glycerin, and potassium sorbate.

Something else to keep in mind about preservatives is the temperature range in which they can be used. When making lotion, for instance, a certain preservative that I've used in the past must be added to the mixture at or below 90°F. (The lotion has to be well above 100 degrees while forming the emulsion.) Unfortunately, it takes over an hour for the lotion to cool down to the appropriate temperature, and this also makes it harder to transfer the lotion into bottles at that point because it gets thicker as it cools.

Antioxidants

If you're going to be using ingredients that are prone to oxidation, such as certain botanical oils, then consider adding one or more antioxidants to your formulation. Popular choices are T-50 vitamin E oil[139] and rosemary oil extract.[140] You can also add a highly stable oil that is naturally high in vitamin E, such as cranberry seed oil.

12

INGREDIENT RESEARCH
TIPS

One of the most frustrating things about DIY anti-aging skin care is that substantiating the claims made by ingredient vendors and companies whose products you wish to imitate often proves difficult. They'll say that such-and-such product "boosts collagen synthesis" or "smooths fine lines and wrinkles," but they don't provide any supporting evidence. Making vague references to "studies" and "clinical trials" without linking to further information is the industry norm, so get used to it.

When you're thinking about using a particular natural ingredient that may contain several bioactive compounds, always ask yourself, "What exactly is it about this material that allegedly produces the desired effects?" A good way to answer this question is to first find out what chemical compounds exist in the material and then research them individually to see if there's any connection between the particular compound and the purported benefits of the material as a whole. That may seem like a tedious and time-consuming process, but unless you make an effort to understand, at the cellular and molecular levels, how such ingredients may or may not affect your skin, you'll be forever at the mercy of charlatans who cherry pick[141] data to advance their agendas and well-meaning people who spread misinformation out of ignorance.

An example of the latter involves rose hip seed oil. On countless websites that discuss its benefits as an anti-aging product, I've seen statements that this oil is rich in vitamin C. This is chemically impossible. As you know, natural vitamin C (L-ascorbic acid) is not soluble in oil; it's soluble in water. Rose hips themselves, however, are known to contain vitamin C, and that's probably the source of the confusion.

So if product vendors, beauty bloggers, and the like are not to be relied upon, how do you find out what chemical substances are in a particular ingredient, and how do you get verifiable proof that a particular ingredient "does what it says on the tin," so to speak? In terms of finding out what's in a multi-compound ingredient, a convenient way to do that is to go to a search engine (Google, Bing, etc.) and use the "right" keywords. It sounds obvious, but it's really not, and it's best explained by example. If, for instance, you wanted to know what's in red raspberry seed oil, you could do the following search:

```
characterization of red raspberry seed oil
```

In the field of analytical chemistry, "characterization" is the process of determining the chemical composition of a substance, including the quantities of individual compounds in the material. Using this technical term in your query is a shortcut to finding the results of professionally conducted research. If you just search for red raspberry seed oil, you'll have to wade through a lot of commercial websites before seeing any scholarly resources.

When looking for professional research studies, there are many other technical terms besides "characterization" that you can use to bypass content whose only purpose is marketing. For example, you can use "epidermis" or "stratum corneum" instead of "skin." If you wanted to find out more about a particular botanical oil, you could search the Latin name of the plant that it comes from instead of the common name (e.g., "*Passiflora edulis*" instead of "maracujá" or "passion fruit").

Another way to find professional research studies is to use the "filetype" command in Google. Many journal articles are published online as PDF documents, and you can access them easily by telling Google that you want to see only files of this type. For example, suppose that you want to know more about topical vitamin C. Rather than just doing a search for "topical vitamin C," it might be more productive to type either of the following in Google's search box:

```
filetype:pdf topical ascorbic acid
topical ascorbic acid filetype:pdf
```

The above searches will show results that are primarily academic, and they should all be PDF files. Yet another shortcut to the good stuff is to use a combination of quotation marks and plus signs. If you wanted information about linoleic acid as it relates to matrix metalloproteinases, you could do the following search:

```
"linoleic acid"+"matrix metalloproteinases"
```

The quotation marks tell Google to return only those results that have the exact word or phrase that you put inside the quotes, while the plus sign indicates that both "linoleic acid" and "matrix metalloproteinases" should be present in each search result. If you did the same search without the quotation marks and plus sign, it wouldn't be as targeted, and you might have to spend several minutes clicking through page after page of results to find the information that you need. In addition to the techniques that I've shown above, there are many other Google search commands[142] that can streamline your searches.

While Google is a good starting point for your research, it's not your only option. PubMed[143] is an excellent search engine for scientific topics, and many of the journal articles that you'll find through that site are available for free. Google Scholar[144] is similar to PubMed, but it's not as good, in my opinion. When you click on an article in PubMed, it will also show you a list of related articles, and this can be a great way to discover more topics and additional research studies whose findings may support or contradict those of whatever study you clicked on first.

If you happen to find papers that are behind a paywall, you can try going to a local university library that is open to the general public. If the school has an extensive collection of academic journals, you'll probably be able to find all of the papers that you want to read, and you can make photocopies of them if necessary, since journals are reference materials that can't be checked out of the library.

13
WHERE TO GET INGREDIENTS

Botanical oils and other skin care ingredients can be purchased at wholesale prices from several online vendors. You're unlikely to find brick-and-mortar retail stores that carry such products, and if you do, the prices will be marked up substantially. On the other hand, the downside to ordering online is the cost of shipping, but sometimes you can get free shipping if your order is above a certain amount. The list of vendors on the following page is by no means comprehensive, but it's enough to get you started.

fromnaturewithlove.com
makingcosmetics.com
lotioncrafter.com
organic-creations.com
wholesalesuppliesplus.com
gardenstatenaturals.com
ingredientstodiefor.com
brambleberry.com

If you're planning to use food-grade botanical oils, you can usually find them online at supplement shops, such as Swanson Vitamins (swansonvitamins.com), as well as directly from the manufacturers (e.g., nutiva.com, nowfoods.com). Health food stores and finer grocery stores are another option, although I would be reluctant to buy oils at either of those places because you never know how long they've been on the shelf. Many of them also come in clear glass bottles. (This is not an issue for coconut oil, which is very stable because of its high saturated fat content.) I recommend buying oils from vendors who understand the importance of proper storage and handling[75] of unrefined botanical oils.

14
WHERE TO GET RECIPES

Thousands of DIY skin care product recipes are waiting for you on the Internet if you know where to look. Among them are plenty of "anti-aging" formulations. For example, MakingCosmetics® (makingcosmetics.com) has an online library of recipes in several product categories, with everything from shampoos to wrinkle creams.

If there's a particular ingredient that you want to use and a particular product that you'd like to make, then a good way to find recipes that use that ingredient is through search engines like DuckDuckGo, Bing, and Google. Let's say that you want to make a face cream

with mango butter. You might do a search in any of the
the above search engines like so:

```
"face cream"+"mango butter"+"recipe"
```

As mentioned in a previous chapter, the quotation
marks ensure that the exact word or phrase inside the
quotes will be in the search results that you get, and the
plus signs indicate that all of the words or phrases that
you've entered will be present in each individual result.
Searching in this very specific way makes it quicker and
easier to find what you're looking for.

Based on my experience, the free recipes that are
available in abundance are "hit or miss," and I usually
end up tweaking them to suit my needs. Sometimes I
come up with a winner, and other times, it's a disaster.
But that's all part of the fun, right?

If there's a commercial product that you really like
and want to make at home, you can search using the
term, "diy copycat," which is part of the lingo of the DIY
skin care community. For example, if you love Burt's
Bees® lip balm, but you don't like paying $3.00 per stick,
then you might search for:

```
burt's bees lip balm diy copycat
```

Lo and behold, someone has done it and shared the recipe with the world.[145]

15
WHERE TO GET EQUIPMENT AND SUPPLIES

Making your own anti-aging skin care products doesn't require any special equipment, with the exception of an accurate digital scale for measuring ingredients. It's best to get a scale that measures to at least two decimal places. Cheap kitchen scales are accurate to only one decimal place, and sometimes an error of a few hundredths of an ounce can make a big difference in the outcome of a recipe. If you can't afford a good scale (the better ones are about $100 or more), then you can try converting the recipe ingredient amounts from ounces to grams. This often results in more favorable numbers that have only one decimal place. (Most kitchen scales allow you to choose whether you want to measure in ounces or grams.) For weighing out ingredients, you can use small, plastic food storage containers, or you can repurpose other types of food containers like yogurt cups.

Other supplies and equipment that you may need are common household items that you probably own already, such as mixing bowls, stirring spoons, measuring spoons, flatware (for scooping and mixing), an electric mixer or hand/stick blender, a wire whisk, rubber spatulas, funnels, an instant-read thermometer, and Pyrex® measuring cups with open handles. A double boiler is helpful, but if you don't have one, then you can create a makeshift double boiler with a saucepan and a Pyrex measuring cup (with the open handle hanging over the side of the saucepan). The Pyrex measuring cups (anywhere from 2-cup to 2-quart in size) can also be used as mixing bowls in procedures that require heat. Regardless of heat requirements, it's best to use mixing bowls that are **non-porous**, **non-reactive**, and **microwave-safe**. Pyrex glass meets all three requirements.

Even though you may already have many of the above items, it's a good idea to have a separate set of bowls, measuring cups, utensils, etc. that you use only for your DIY skin care projects so that you don't run the risk of contaminating the same ones that are used for eating or preparing food. These items can be picked up cheaply at Walmart, Dollar General, and similar places. Thrift shops and yard sales are great options, too.

For storing your finished products, you can purchase the appropriate containers or reuse the ones from cosmetics and toiletries that you already have, as long as you clean, sterilize, and label them. While new bottles, tins, and other containers tend to be inexpensive, there may be a minimum order requirement if you purchase them from online shops that specialize in containers. If there's no minimum, then expect to pay upwards of $10.00 to ship a little plastic jar that costs a buck.

One way to save money on containers is to order them from the same companies that sell the ingredients that you're buying. Another way to save money on containers is to go to a dollar store and purchase some cheap products that come in the types of containers that you want. Empty the containers, and clean them thoroughly with hot water and dish soap. Be sure to sterlize them just before use by soaking them in a water-and-bleach solution for a few minutes, followed by rinsing them with water and allowing the containers to air-dry on a clean surface. Do the same for any other items that will come into contact with your product during preparation, such as spoons, mixing bowls, spatulas, etc.

16
WHERE TO GET EDUCATED

When looking for recipes, you may discover that some publishers assume a level of technical knowledge that you may or may not have. If you want to make a lotion, for example, you'll need to know about emulsions[146] and how they're formed, but if the recipe doesn't offer detailed, step-by-step instructions for the benefit of a beginner, then you may not be able to proceed. Knowing the purpose of each ingredient would be useful as well. The following resources can help you learn how to make specific types of products and understand the science behind them.

MakingCostmetics® Resources[147]
Lotioncrafter® Reference Room[148]

Lotioncrafter® Books[149]
From Nature With Love® Bookstore[150]
Cosmetics & Toiletries: Science Applied[151]
Alluredbooks: Specialty Science Books[152]

REFERENCES

All URLs (shown in italics) were valid at the time of publishing. If any website document listed below is no longer available, then you can try using the "WayBack Machine" to find the missing content. Go to **https://archive.org/** and enter the URL of the document of interest into the WayBack Machine search box. If the old content has been archived, then you'll be presented with a list of dates on which a "snap shot" was taken of that particular URL. Click on a date to see what the page looked like at that time.

1. What People Are Saying.
   http://www.realhandmadesoap.com/folders/What%20people%20are%20saying.htm

2. The Relevance of High SPF Products: High SPF Sunscreens Help Compensate Under-Application.
   http://www.neutrogenamd.com/text/content/downloads/Ouyang_2011_HighSPF.pdf

3. The Electromagnetic Spectrum.
   http://imagine.gsfc.nasa.gov/science/toolbox/emspectrum1.html

4. Sunscreen: The Burning Facts.
   http://www.epa.gov/sunwise/doc/sunscreen.pdf

5. Goh EG, Xu X, McCormick PG. 2014. Effect of particle size on the UV absorbance of zinc oxide nanoparticles. Scripta Mater. 78-79:49-52.

6. Nusgens BV, Humbert P, Rougier A, Richard A, Lapière CM. 2002. Stimulation of collagen biosynthesis by topically applied vitamin C. Eur J Dermatol. 12(4):XXXII-XXXIV.

7. Nusgens BV, Humbert P, Rougier A, Colige AC, Haftek M, Lambert CA, Richard A, Creidi P, Lapière CM. 2001. Topically applied vitamin C enhances the mRNA level of collagens I and III, their processing enzymes and tissue inhibitor of matrix metalloproteinase 1 in the human dermis. J Invest Dermatol. 116(6):853-9.

8. Haftek M, Creidi P, Richard A, Humbert P, Schmitt D, Rougier A. 2002. Topically applied ascorbic acid helps to restructure chronically photodamaged human skin. Eur J Dermatol. 12(4):XXVII-XXIX.

9. Humbert PG, Haftek M, Creidi P, Lapière C, Nusgens B, Richard A, Schmitt D, Rougier A, Zahouani H. 2003. Topical ascorbic acid on photoaged skin. Clinical, topographical and ultrastructural evaluation: double-blind study vs. placebo. Exp Dermatol. 12(3):237-44.

10. Darr D, Combs S, Dunston S, Manning T, Pinnell S. 1992. Topical vitamin C protects porcine skin from ultraviolet radiation-induced damage. Br J Dermatol. 127(3):247-53.

11. Plasencia I, Norlén L, Bagatolli LA. 2007. Direct visualization of lipid domains in human skin stratum corneum's lipid membranes: effect of pH and temperature. Biophys J. 93(9):3142-55.

12. Barba C, Martí M, Semenzato A, Baratto G, Manich AM, Coderch L. 2015. Effect of lipid modification on stratum corneum permeability. J. Therm. Anal. Calorim. 120(1):297-305.

13. Pinnell SR, Yang H, Omar M, Riviere NM, DeBuys HV, Walker LC, Wang Y, Levine M. 2001. Topical L-Ascorbic Acid: Percutaneous Absorption Studies. Dermatol Surg. 27(2):137-142.

14. Lin FH, Lin JY, Gupta RD, Tournas JA, Burch JA, Selim MA, Monteiro-Riviere NA, Grichnik JM, Zielinski J, Pinnell SR. 2005. Ferulic acid stabilizes a solution of vitamins C and E and doubles its photoprotection of skin. J Invest Dermatol. 125(4):826-32.

15. Pinnell SR, Yang H, Omar M, Riviere NM, DeBuys HV, Walker LC, Wang Y, Levine M. 2001. Topical L-Ascorbic Acid: Percutaneous Absorption Studies. Dermatol Surg. 27(2):137-142.

16. Traikovich SS. 1999. Use of topical ascorbic acid and its effects on photodamaged skin typography. Ama Arch Otolaryngol. 25(10):1091-1098.

17. Meves A, Stock SN, Beyerle A, Pittelkow MR, Peus D. 2002. Vitamin C derivative ascorbyl palmitate promotes ultraviolet-B-induced lipid peroxidation and cytotoxicity in keratinocytes. J Invest Dermatol. 119:1103-1108.

18. Geesin JC, Gordon JS, Berg RA. 1993. Regulation of collagen synthesis in human dermal fibroblasts by the sodium and magnesium salts of ascorbyl-2-phosphate. Skin Pharmacol. 6(1):65-71.

19. Davidson JM, LuValle PA, Zoia O, Quaglino D Jr, Giro M. 1997. Ascorbate differentially regulates elastin and collagen biosynthesis in vascular smooth muscle cells and skin fibroblasts by pretranslational mechanisms. J Biol Chem. 272(1):345-52.

20. Rhie GE, Shin MH, Seo JY, Choi WW, Cho KH, Kim KH, Park KC, Eun HC, Chung JH. 2001. Aging- and photoaging-dependent changes of enzymic and nonenzymic antioxidants in the epidermis and dermis of human skin in vivo. J Invest Dermatol. 117:1212–1217.

21. Lévèque N, Robin S, Makki S, Muret P, Rougier A, Humbert P. 2003. Iron and ascorbic acid concentrations in human dermis with regard to age and body sites. Gerontology. 49(2):117-22.

22. Lévèque N, Muret P, Mary S, Makki S, Kantelip JP, Rougier A, Humbert P. 2002. Decrease in skin ascorbic acid concentration with age. Eur J Dermatol. 12(4):XXI-XXII.

23. Pinnell SR, Madey DL. 1999. The benefits of topical vitamin C (L-ascorbic acid) for skin care and UV protection. J Appl Cosmetol. 18:126-134.

24. Lin JY, Selim MA, Shea CR, Grichnik JM, Omar MM, Monteiro-Riviere NA, Pinnell SR. 2003. UV photoprotection by combination topical antioxidants vitamin C and vitamin E. J Am Acad Dermatol. 48:866–874.

25. Brown MW. 2003. Antioxidants – what is their significance in sun protection? SÖFW Journal. 129(7):2-12.

26. Wu G, Fang YZ, Yang S, Lupton JR, Turner ND. 2004. Glutathione metabolism and its implications for health. J Nutr. 134(3):489-492.

27. Quan T, Qin Z, Xia W, Shao Y, Voorhees JJ, Fisher GJ. 2009. Matrix-degrading metalloproteinases in photoaging. J Invest Dermatol. 14:20-24.

28. Simopoulos AP. 2003. Importance of the ratio of omega-6/omega-3 essential fatty acids: evolutionary aspects. World Rev Nutr Diet. 92:1-22.

29. Simopoulos AP. 2002. The importance of the ratio of omega-6/omega-3 essential fatty acids. Biomed Pharmacother. 56(8):365-79.

30. Simopoulos AP. 2008. The omega-6/omega-3 fatty acid ratio, genetic variation, and cardiovascular disease. Asia Pac J Clin Nutr. 17 Suppl 1:131-4.

31. Precious Yet Perilous.
http://www.westonaprice.org/health-topics/precious-yet-perilous/

32. Ziboh VA, Miller CC, Cho Y. 2000. Metabolism of polyunsaturated fatty acids by skin epidermal enzymes: generation of antiinflammatory and antiproliferative metabolites. Am J Clin Nutr. 71(1):361s-366s.

33. Hansen HS, Jensen B. 1985. Essential function of linoleic acid esterified in acylglucosylceramide and acylceramide in maintaining the epidermal water permeability barrier. Evidence from feeding studies with oleate, linoleate, arachidonate, columbinate and alpha-linolenate. Biochim Biophys Acta. 834(3):357-63.

34. Skolnik P, Eaglstein WH, Ziboh VA. 1977. Human essential fatty acid deficiency: treatment by topical application of linoleic acid. Arch Dermatol. 113(7):939-41.

35. Press M, Hartop PJ, Prottey C. 1974. Correction of essential fatty-acid deficiency in man by the cutaneous application of sunflower-seed oil. Lancet. 303(7858):597-599.

36. Burdge GC, Wootton SA. 2002. Conversion of alpha-linolenic acid to eicosapentaenoic, docosapentaenoic and docosahexaenoic acids in young women. Br J Nutr. 88(4):411-20.

37. Kim HH, Shin CM, Park C, Kim KH, Cho KH, Eun HC, Chung JH. 2005. Eicosapentaenoic acid inhibits UV-induced MMP-1 expression in human dermal fibroblasts. J Lipid Res. 46:1712-1720.

38. Kim HH, Cho S, Lee S, Kim KH, Cho KH, Eun HC, Chung JH. 2006. Photoprotective and anti-skin-aging effects of eicosapentaenoic acid in human skin in vivo. J Lipid Res. 47(5):921-30.

39. Moison RM, Steenvoorden DP, Beijersbergen van Henegouwen GM. 2001. Topically applied eicosapentaenoic acid protects against local immunosuppression induced by UVB irradiation, cis-urocanic acid and thymidine dinucleotides. Photochem Photobiol. 73(1):64-70.

40. Moison RM, Beijersbergen Van Henegouwen GM. 2001. Dietary eicosapentaenoic acid prevents systemic immunosuppression in mice induced by UVB radiation. Radiat Res. 156(1):36-44.

41. Rhodes LE, O'Farrell S, Jackson MJ, Friedmann PS. 1994. Dietary fish-oil supplementation in humans reduces UVB-erythemal sensitivity but increases epidermal lipid peroxidation. J Invest Dermatol. 103(2):151-4.

42. Meydani M, Natiello F, Goldin B, Free N, Woods M, Schaefer E, Blumberg JB, Gorback SL. 1991. Effect of long-term fish oil supplementation on vitamin E status and lipid peroxidation in women. J Nutr. 121(4):484-491.

43. Pilkington SM, Watson RE, Nicolaou A, Rhodes LE. 2011. Omega-3 polyunsaturated fatty acids: photoprotective macronutrients. Exp Dermatol. 20(7):537-543.

44. Sies H, Stahl W. 2004. Nutritional protection against skin damage from sunlight. Annu Rev Nutr. 24:173-200.

45. Fernández-García E. 2014. Skin protection against UV light by dietary antioxidants. Food Funct. 5(9):1994-2003.

46. Heinrich U, Neukam K, Tronnier H, Sies H, Stahl W. 2006. Long-term ingestion of high flavanol cocoa provides photoprotection against UV-induced erythema and improves skin condition in women. J Nutr. 136(6):1565-9.

47. Stahl W, Heinrich U, Aust O, Tronnier H, Sies H. 2006. Lycopene-rich products and dietary photoprotection. Photochem Photobiol Sci. 5(2):238-42.

48. Hassan I, Dorjay K, Sami A, Anwar P. 2013. Sunscreens and antioxidants as photoprotective measures: an update. Our Dermatol Online. 4(3):369-374.

49. Kligman LH, Akin FJ, Kligman AM. 1983. Sunscreens promote repair of ultraviolet radiation-induced dermal damage. J Invest Dermatol. 81:98-102.

50. Ando H, Ryu A, Hashimoto A, Oka M, Ichihashi M. 1998. Linoleic acid and alpha-linolenic acid lightens ultraviolet-induced hyperpigmentation of the skin. Arch Dermatol Res. 290(7):375-81.

51. Harrison C. 2014. Patenting natural products just got harder. Nature Biotechnol. 32:403-404.

52. The Patent Office Clarifies the Ban on Patenting Naturally-Derived Drugs and Other Products.
    http://www.jdsupra.com/legalnews/the-patent-office-clarifies-the-ban-on-p-34356/

53. Can You Patent a Natural Product? Prepare for a Different Answer.
    http://pipeline.corante.com/archives/2014/04/08/can_you_patent_a_natural_product_prepare_for_a_different_answer.php

54. Why Natural Products?
    http://www.scripps.edu/shen/NPLI/whynaturalproducts.html

55. Like Dissolves Like and Molecule Ion Attractions.
    http://www.kentchemistry.com/links/bonding/LikeDissolveslike.htm

56. Ester.
    http://en.wikipedia.org/wiki/Ester

57. Humectant.
    http://en.wikipedia.org/wiki/Humectant

58. Ebling FJ. 1965. The sebaceous glands. J Soc Cosmetic Chemists. 16:405-411.

59. Andiroba Oil, Refined.
    http://www.naturalsourcing.com/product-literature/NS_info_andiroba_oil.pdf

60. Cabrera-Vique C, Marfil R, Giménez R, Martínez-Augustin O. 2012. Bioactive compounds and nutritional significance of virgin argan oil - an edible oil with potential as a functional food. Nutr Rev. 70(5):266-279.

61. Khallouki F, Younos C, Soulimani R, Oster T, Charrouf Z, Spiegelhalder B, Bartsch H, Owen RW. 2003. Consumption of argan oil (Morocco) with its unique profile of fatty acids, tocopherols, squalene, sterols and phenolic compounds should confer valuable cancer chemopreventive effects. Eur J Cancer Prev. 12(1):67-75.

62. Virgin Organic Argan Oil (Deodorized).
    http://www.naturalsourcing.com/product-literature/NS_info_arganOil.pdf

63. Avocado Oil.
    http://www.naturalsourcing.com/product-literature/NS_info_AvocadoOil.pdf

64. Baobab Oil Classic Cold Pressed Organic - For Cosmetics
    Formulations.
    *http://www.baobabfruitco.com/Products/BaobabOils/BaobabOilOrganicColdPr
    essed.html*

65. Extra Pure Baobab Oil.
    http://www.baobabfruitco.com/pdf/Pdf/ExtraPureBaobabOil.pdf

66. Baobab Oil Unrefined.
    http://www.naturalsourcing.com/spec/SPEC_Baobab_Oil_Unrefined.pdf

67. Bushman BS, Phillips B, Isbell T, Ou BX, Crane JM, Knapp, SJ. 2004.
    Chemical composition of caneberry (Rubus spp.) seeds and oils and
    their antioxidant potential. J Agr Food Chem. 52(26):7982-7987.

68. Blackberry Seed Oil.
    http://www.naturalsourcing.com/spec/SPEC_Blackberry_Seed_Oil.pdf

69. Dulf FV, Bele C, Unguresan M, Parlog R, Socaciu C. 2009.
    Phytosterols as markers in identification of the adulterated pumpkin
    seed oil with sunflower oil. Bull Univ Agric Sci. 66(2):301-307.

70. Rapid Measurement of Olive Oil Adulteration with Seed Oils with
    Minimal Sample Preparation Using DSA/TOF.
    *http://www.perkinelmer.com/CMSResources/Images/44-
    161678APP_OliveOilAdulteration.pdf*

71. Detection of Adulterant Seed Oils in Extra Virgin Olive Oils by LC-
    MS and Principal Components Analysis.
    *http://www.absciex.com/Documents/Downloads/Literature/mass-spectrometry-
    Adultaration-OliveOil-1282510.pdf*

72. Van Hoed V, Barbouche I, De Clercq N, Dewettinck K, Slah M, Leber E, Verhé R. 2011. Influence of filtering of cold pressed berry seed oils on their antioxidant profile and quality characteristics. Food Chem. 127(4):1848-1855.

73. Value-Adding Factors in Cold-Pressed Edible Seed Oils and Flours. *http://drum.lib.umd.edu/bitstream/1903/4173/1/umi-umd-3974.pdf*

74. Vegetable Oil Storage Tips and Guidelines. *http://fromnaturewithlove.com/library/storagevegetableoils.asp*

75. Blueberry Seed Oil. *http://www.naturalsourcing.com/downloads/spec/SPEC_Blueberry_Seed_Oil.pdf*

76. Horrobin DF. 1993. Fatty acid metabolism in health and disease: the role of delta-6-desaturase. Am J Clin Nutr. 57(5):732S-736S.

77. Horrobin DF. 1981. Loss of delta-6-desaturase activity as a key factor in aging. Med Hypotheses. 7(9):1211-20.

78. Brosche T, Platt D. 2000. Effect of borage oil consumption on fatty acid metabolism, transepidermal water loss and skin parameters in elderly people. Arch Gerontol Geriat. 30(2):139-150.

79. Organic Borage Oil (20% GLA). *http://www.naturalsourcing.com/spec/SPEC_Organic_Borage_Oil.pdf*

80. Characterisation of Borage Oil by GC-MS. *http://citeseerx.ist.psu.edu/viewdoc/summary?doi=10.1.1.219.5661*

81. How to Use Japanese Camellia Oil. *http://wawaza.com/pages/How-to-Use-Japanese-Camellia-%28Tsubaki%29-Oil.html*

82. Pazyar N, Yaghoobi R, Bagherani N, Kazerouni A. 2013. A review of applications of tea tree oil in dermatology. Int J Dermatol. 52(7):784-90.

83. Tsubaki (Camellia japonica) cold-pressed oil: composition, protection from oxidation and moisturizing properties.
http://www.researchgate.net/publication/268219763_Tsubaki_%28Camellia_ja ponica%29_cold-pressed_oil_composition_protection_from_oxidation_and_ moisturizing_properties

84. Cold Pressed Carrot Seed Oil.
http://www.naturalsourcing.com/product.asp?product_id=OILCARROTCPUS5 74

85. Nawar, Wassef W. Cranberry seed oil extract and compositions containing components thereof.
https://www.google.com/patents/US7517540

86. Van Hoed V, De Clercq N, Echim C, Andjelkovic M, Leber E, Dewettinck K, Verhe R. 2009. Berry seeds: a source of specialty oils with high content of bioactives and nutritional value. J Food Lipids. 16(1):33-49.

87. Cucumber Seed Oil.
https://www.naturalsourcing.com/downloads/newsmedia/CucumberSeedOil_N S_082712.pdf

88. Organic Evening Primrose Oil 10% GLA Min.
http://www.naturalsourcing.com/downloads/spec/SPEC_Organic_Evening_Pri mrose_Oil_10_GLA.pdf

89. Canbay HS, Bardakçı B. 2011. Determination of fatty acid, C, H, N and trace element composition in grape seed by GC/MS, FTIR, elemental analyzer and ICP/OES. SDU Journal of Science. 6(2):140-148.

90. Chilean Hazelnut Oil (Gevuina).
http://www.naturalsourcing.com/spec/SPEC_Chilean_Hazelnut_CP.pdf

91. Hazelnut Oil.
http://www.naturalsourcing.com/spec/SPEC_Hazelnut_Oil.pdf

92. Wille JJ, Kydonieus A. 2003. Palmitoleic acid isomer (C16:1delta6) in human skin sebum is effective against gram-positive bacteria. Skin Pharmacol Appl Skin Physiol. 16(3):176-87.

93. Russo, Ethan B. 2002. Cannabis and Cannabinoids: Pharmacology, Toxicology, and Therapeutic Potential. Binghamton (NY): The Haworth Press, Inc. p. 423.

94. Chen T, He J, Zhang J, Zhang H, Qian P, Hao J, Li L. 2010. Analytical characterization of Hempseed (seed of Cannabis sativa L.) oil from eight regions in China. J Diet Suppl. 7(2):117-29.

95. Organic Cold-Pressed Hemp Oil.
   https://store.nutiva.com/cold-pressed-hemp-oil/

96. Nutritional Composition of Hemp Seed and Oil.
   http://nutiva.com/wp-content/uploads/2011/11/Hemp-Compositon-Chart1.pdf

97. Horrobin DF, Manku MS. 1989. Premenstrual syndrome and premenstrual breast pain (cyclical mastalgia): disorders of essential fatty acid (EFA) metabolism. Prostag Leukotr Ess. 37(4):255-261.

98. Kim EJ, Kim MK, Jin XJ, Oh JH, Kim JE, Chung JH. 2010. Skin aging and photoaging alter fatty acids composition, including 11,14,17-eicosatrienoic acid, in the epidermis of human skin. J Korean Med Sci. 25(6):980-3.

99. Haze S, Gozu Y, Nakamura S, Kohno Y, Sawano K, Ohta H, Yamazaki K. 2001. 2-Nonenal newly found in human body odor tends to increase with aging. J Invest Dermatol. 116(4):520-4.

100. Virgin Macadamia Nut Oil.
   http://www.naturalsourcing.com/spec/SPEC_Macadamia_Nut_Oil_Virgin.pdf

101. Malacrida CS, Jorge N. 2012. Yellow Passion Fruit Seed Oil (Passiflora edulis f. flavicarpa): Physical and Chemical Characteristics. Braz Arch Biol Techn. 55(1):127-134.

102. Matsui Y1, Sugiyama K, Kamei M, Takahashi T, Suzuki T, Katagata Y, Ito T. 2010. Extract of passion fruit (Passiflora edulis) seed containing high amounts of piceatannol inhibits melanogenesis and promotes collagen synthesis. J Agric Food Chem. 58(20):11112-11118.

103. Jorge AT, Arroteia KF, Santos IA, Andres E, Medina SP, Ferrari CR, Lourenço CB, Biaggio RM, Moreira PL. 2012. Schinus terebinthifolius Raddi extract and linoleic acid from Passiflora edulis synergistically decrease melanin synthesis in B16 cells and reconstituted epidermis. Int J Cosmet Sci. 34(5):435-40.

104. Maracuja Oil.
http://tartecosmetics.com/tarte-item-pure-maracuja-oil

105. Maracuja (Passionfruit) Oil, Virgin.
https://www.fromnaturewithlove.com/soap/product.asp?product_id=OILMARA EXPVIRPR664

106. Chemistry of New Industrial Oil Seed Crops.
http://www.hort.purdue.edu/newcrop/proceedings1990/V1-196.html

107. Burg DA, Kleiman R. 1991. Preparation of meadowfoam dimer acids and dimer esters, and their use as lubricants. J Am Oil Chem Soc. 68(8):600-603.

108. A Comparison of Meadowfoam Seed Oil and Jojoba Oil.
http://www.elementis.com/esweb/webprodliterature.nsf/allbydocid/81C33FD0B 999EA5585257AAA00544468/$FILE/meadowfoam%20comparison7-13.pdf

109. Isbell TA, Abbott TP, Carlson KD. 1999. Oxidative stability index of vegetable oils in binary mixtures with meadowfoam oil. Ind Crop Prod. 9(2):115-123.

110. Basic Report: 11222, Drumstick leaves, raw.
http://ndb.nal.usda.gov/ndb/foods/show/3009

111. Cater NB, Denke MA. 2001. Behenic acid is a cholesterol-raising saturated fatty acid in humans. Am J Clin Nutr. 73(1):41-44.

112. Lalas S, Tsaknis J. 2002. Characterization of Moringa oleifera seed oil variety "Periyakulam 1". J Food Compos Anal. 15:65-77.

113. Rashid U, Anwar F, Moser BR, Knothe G. 2008. Moringa oleifera oil: a possible source of biodiesel. Bioresour Technol. 99(17):8175-9.

114. Aslam MN, Lansky EP, Varani J. 2006. Pomegranate as a cosmeceutical source: pomegranate fractions promote proliferation and procollagen synthesis and inhibit matrix metalloproteinase-1 production in human skin cells. J Ethnopharmacol. 103(3):311-8.

115. Grossmann ME, Mizuno NK, Schuster T, Cleary MP. 2010. Punicic acid is an ω-5 fatty acid capable of inhibiting breast cancer proliferation. Int J Oncol. 36(2):421-426.

116. About Berry Beautiful.
http://www.berrybeautiful.us/about-us.html

117. Oomah BD, Ladet S, Godfrey DV, Liang J, Girard B. 2000. Characteristics of raspberry (Rubus idaeus L.) seed oil. Food Chem. 69(2):187-193.

118. Red Raspberry Seed Oil.
http://www.naturalsourcing.com/downloads/spec/SPEC_Red_Raspberry_Seed_Oil.pdf

119. Xu Z, Samuel Godber JS. 1999. Purification and identification of components of γ-oryzanol in rice bran oil. J Agric Food Chem. 47(7):2724–2728.

120. Rogers EJ, Rice SM, Nicolosi RJ, Carpenter DR, McClelland CA, Romanczyk Jr, LJ. 1993. Identification and quantitation of γ-oryzanol components and simultaneous assessment of tocols in rice bran oil. J Am Oil Chem Soc. 70(3):301-307.

121. Scavariello EM, Arellano DB. 1998. Gamma-oryzanol: an important component in rice brain oil. Arch Latinoam Nutr. 48(1):7-12.

122. Xu Z, Hua N, Godber JS. 2001. Antioxidant activity of tocopherols, tocotrienols, and gamma-oryzanol components from rice bran against cholesterol oxidation accelerated by 2,2'-azobis(2-methylpropionamidine) dihydrochloride. J Agric Food Chem. 49(4):2077-81.

123. Sugano M, Tsuji E. 1997. Rice bran oil and cholesterol metabolism. J Nutr. 127(3):5215-5245.

124. Most MM, Tulley R, Morales S, Lefevre M. 2005. Rice bran oil, not fiber, lowers cholesterol in humans. Am J Clin Nutr. 81(1):64-68.

125. Ishihara M, Ito Y, Nakakita T, Maehama T, Hieda S, Yamamoto K, Ueno N. 1982. Clinical effect of gamma-oryzanol on climacteric disturbance on serum lipid peroxides. Nihon Sanka Fujinka Gakkai Zasshi. 34(2):243-51.

126. Kaewkool P. 2011. Characterization of cold pressed organic rice bran oil. As J Food Ag-Ind. 4(1):16-21.

127. Concha J, Soto C, Chamy R, Zúñiga ME. 2006. Effect of rosehip extraction process on oil and defatted meal physicochemical properties. J Am Oil Chem Soc. 83(9):771-775.

128. Tretinoin (Topical Route).
http://www.mayoclinic.org/drugs-supplements/tretinoin-topical-route/description/drg-20066521

129. Yang B, Kallio HP. 2001. Fatty acid composition of lipids in sea buckthorn (Hippophaë rhamnoides L.) berries of different origins. J Agric Food Chem. 49(4):1939-47.

130. Zeb A. 2004. Chemical and nutritional constituents of sea buckthorn juice. Pakistan J Nutr. 3(2):99-106.

131. Seglina D, Karklina D, Ruisa S, Krasnova I. 2006. The effect of processing on the composition of sea buckthorn juice. J Fruit Ornam Plant Res. 14(Suppl. 2):257-264.

132. Larmo, Petra. The Health Effects of Sea Buckthorn Berries and Oil.
http://www.doria.fi/bitstream/handle/10024/66646/Larmo_DISS1.pdf

133. Luo CX, Zhang GD, Chen R. 2006. Fatty acid compositions of strawberry seed oil. China Oils and Fats. Issue 5:(68-69).

134. Coconut Oil.
https://en.wikipedia.org/wiki/Coconut_oil

135. Baobab Oil Unrefined.
http://www.naturalsourcing.com/spec/SPEC_Baobab_Oil_Unrefined.pdf

136. Volume Conversion.
http://www.metric-conversions.org/volume-conversion.htm

137. Lincoln Fine Ingredients: Products.
http://www.chemteccc.com/pages/lincoln_prds.html

138. Linatural.
http://www.organic-creations.com/preservatives/466-linatural

139. Vitamin E, Mixed Tocopherols T50.
http://www.lotioncrafter.com/mixed-tocopherols-t50-natural-vitamin-e.html

140. Rosemary Oleoresin Extract (ROE).
http://www.lotioncrafter.com/rosemary-oleoresin-roe.html

141. Cherry Picking Fallacy.
http://en.wikipedia.org/wiki/Cherry_picking_%28fallacy%29

142. Google Power User Tips: Query Operators.
http://searchengineland.com/google-power-user-tips-query-operators-48126

143. PubMed.
http://www.ncbi.nlm.nih.gov/pubmed/

144. Google Scholar.
https://scholar.google.com/

145. Burts Bees Lip Balm Recipe {Copy Cat}.
http://happymoneysaver.com/burts-bees-lip-balm-recipe/

146. Emulsions and the HMB System.
http://www.lotioncrafter.com/pdf/Emulsions_&_HLB_System.pdf

147. MakingCostmetics® Resources.
http://www.makingcosmetics.com/Resources_ep_41.html

148. Lotioncrafter® Reference Room.
http://www.lotioncrafter.com/lotioncrafter-premium-ingredients-reference-room.html

149. Lotioncrafter® Books.
   http://www.lotioncrafter.com/lotioncrafter-premium-ingredients-books/

150. From Nature With Love® Bookstore.
   http://fromnaturewithlove.com/bookstore/viewall.asp

151. Cosmetics & Toiletries: Science Applied.
   http://www.cosmeticsandtoiletries.com/

152. Alluredbooks: Specialty Science Books.
   http://www.alluredbooks.com/

153. Yes – Fats Can Be Healthy for You!
   http://www.drsalzarulo.com/client-handouts/Healthy_Fats.pdf